Night Time Shadows

"Patrick's Story"

By

Margaret Ann Foster BSc (Hons)

ISBN-13: 9781507760574
ISBN-10: 1507760574

Contact
margaretfosterauthor@gmail.com

Dedication

To You Dad

Introduction

Over fifteen years my father Patrick came to terms with and fought off the different stages of Parkinson's disease, along with many other illnesses which often go hand in glove with the disease. As his condition progressed, and we became involved, the path this disease led us along became a learning curve for us all. Often there were times when a solution to an individual problem was not readily apparent, meaning that a process of trial and error had to be employed. During these moments of uncertainty, indecision and insecurity, Patrick showed an immense strength of character in his approach to what is a cruel illness. Although there were times when he could not understand what was happening to him, or why; he never really complained about anything as he fought the challenging experiences the changing years brought with them. Many of the professional members of the medical teams, who had occasion to treat Patrick, were quick to comment on how gentlemanly his manner was, and how easy he was to treat. He was not just a patient to them, he was a friend, and everyone remembers him for his cheeky grin and his cheerful wave goodbye.

In the last few years of his illness, when I was fortunate enough to attend university and read for a degree in psychological studies, my father's fortitude and determination played no small part in providing the inspiration for my final year's dissertation, which was entitled "Who Cares." Unlike our situation, caring for someone with Parkinson's tends to fall upon the shoulders of an aging generation, and so my dissertation considered the plight of spouses who are faced with looking after a partner with Parkinson's. For those who may be interested in a more academic outlook on the subject, at the end of my father's story I have taken the opportunity to include some excerpts which I hope will build a background to this unrelenting condition. There is also a comprehensive bibliography and I would like to acknowledge and thank all these authors for the extensive research they have made available.

There have been books written about the disease itself, and also books from a caring point of view, but Parkinson's varies tremendously from person to person; and it is often said that the symptoms of no two people are ever alike. This book is written through Patrick's eyes, and tells the story of a Parkinson's sufferer from the onset. Although my father did not put pen to paper, after spending eleven years of living together and caring for him, I can say that my husband Geoff and I knew my father very well. We have talked and listened to him throughout his journey and have been beside him every step of the way. For us, the last eleven years have been far from doom and gloom; they have been an education and a privilege.

This is his story.

Margaret.

Chapter One

(2010)

'Happy birthday Dad, do you know how old you are today?'

I attempt to speak, but I can't. I try again, but only the slightest of whispers come out. Margaret doesn't hear me, and patiently leans forward and asks me to say it again. After the third endeavour, I have forgotten what I was going to say anyway!

'You're eighty three today, happy birthday.'

I nod. That's the most I can do until my tablets start to kick in. Neither can I smile, not yet, not until my facial muscles start to work. Some days the tablets can take up to an hour before they have any kind of effect. If I make a real effort I can throw my voice with one loud shout, but the times I really want to shout out are when I have the nightmares that haunt me; although they are not nightmares . . . they are real. Don't you have to be sleeping to have nightmares? I see dead people during the night. Some I recognise and some I don't. They frighten me and I can't shout for help. Shadows lurk in the corners waiting for me, and sometimes a shadow will hover over my bed and I hit out, fighting it off me. Tall shadows, dressed in long coats with a trilby hat tipped over their faces, and some are wearing hooded cloaks, leaning over my bed. I cannot shout for help, even though the baby alarm is connected to the landing upstairs, no-one can hear me.

I wish I was in my old bed upstairs again. My bedroom downstairs is very modern and it's a bright sunny room during the day, but I feel isolated at night, especially as I cannot sleep. I try to make a noise by rattling the metal sides of my bed, you know the sort I mean . . . *cot rails.* I cannot sit up without help, nor can I turn over in bed once I'm in a prone position. Although I can move about a little during the day, when I am laying down I have no choice but to stay where I am, unless I'm moved by Margaret or

Geoff. I'm a man trapped in a body where the muscles have gone into retirement.

The shadows were so frightening one night that, using all my strength, I rattled the rails as hard as I could. Margaret came downstairs to find me distressed and I told her in the slightest of whispers, but with all the effort I could muster.

'There are people in my room and shadows. The shadows are trying to get me. Look, over there.' I say, pointing to the corner of the room, but the shadows have gone now. Margaret touches my hand and tries to reassure me.

'I know they seem real to you, Dad, but it's only because you're half asleep and half awake. The mind plays tricks when you're tired and the medication doesn't help either . . . what's that on your face?'

'I didn't do it,' I try to say. 'It was them. I had a fight with one of them and he scratched me.'

But she cannot hear me.

'It looks as if you've scratched yourself. I'll cut your nails in the morning. It's much better in here with this nightlight, isn't it?'

She kisses my forehead and goes back to bed. My eyes scan around the edges of the room. The shadows have gone . . . for tonight anyway.

Chapter Two

Life without Joyce

(1997)

Sitting at the side of my lovely wife of fifty years, I gently hold on to her hand as she drifts in and out of consciousness. Her face changes from a peaceful look of serenity and then distorts, as once more the medication loses its power to help with the pain.

Joyce knew she had cancer long before the doctors and specialists confirmed their findings. Cancer is a pitiless disease, as most people who have watched a loved one pass away after weeks and months of agonising pain, know only too well. Unfortunately, for Joyce, it was made worse because the medical profession didn't take the time to listen to her. She had been repeatedly told by her GPs that she was suffering from both Arthritis and Irritable Bowel Syndrome, until eventually the day came when the specialist told her it was cancer. Almost instantly a look of relief spread over her face. Not that for one minute was she glad to hear she had cancer, but for a doctor to finally believe the pain she was suffering, was as severe as she said it was, came as a kind of relief. At last a doctor finally believed her. I will never forget the words that were said on that terrible day.

'I'm sorry, but the results from the tests we carried out confirm you have cancer Mrs Millar, and unfortunately it has spread. We will start you on morphine shortly, which should help with the pain.'

Joyce was so composed it broke my heart.

'Now you know its cancer, will you be able to cure it doctor?' she asked the cancer consultant. 'Will you be able to operate, or will I have chemotherapy?'

'Unfortunately no, we can't operate and it's too advanced for chemotherapy . . . but we will do all we can to make you comfortable, and we can send you to Weston Park Hospital where they have better equipment and . . . '

The consultant looked uneasy at being asked such a question, and Joyce and I then realised the cancer must be terminal. There were eight people in the room, including my five children, Margaret, the eldest, Teresa, Patrick, Tony and Kevin, the youngest, and of course the consultant. The room went silent and Joyce stared at the floor for a few minutes, deep in thought, and I suppose in shock. We were all afraid to ask how long she had left to live. But as usual, Joyce was more concerned about the effect it would have on me, our five children and all of our grandchildren. I tried hard to fight back the tears that welled in my throat until I thought I would choke. Our sons and daughters left the room to give us a bit of privacy, and I suppose to let go of their own emotions. Joyce reached up and kissed me as my tears fell on her cheek.

'Don't be upset Paddy. I'm sixty eight years old. I've had my life. I've seen my kids grow up, and their kids; and I've been lucky enough to see two great grandchildren come into the world. I'm not afraid of dying . . . not after living these last six months in pain like this. I've had enough Paddy. I can't take anymore, and anyway, death is only like going through one door into another room. I'll get to see me mam and dad, and our Tom. I know they will be waiting for me.' She said calmly, trying to reassure me as always. 'I've had a happy life with you Paddy. I want you to know that. Don't be upset. We all have to die at some time . . . aw come here. Don't cry Paddy.'

I bent down to her face and she reached up to kiss me once more, her frail body so racked with pain, that I couldn't even hold her. That was the last real kiss we ever had. Within a few weeks the cancer spread rapidly throughout her whole body. Now she was going to die.

I had a strange experience just after Joyce died. When someone you love is in a hospital bed dying from cancer, there isn't much time to think, especially in Joyce's case where the diagnosis was only a matter of weeks before she died. Your only concern is being by their side and doing the best you can to comfort them. On the day they pass away, funeral plans have to be made. The family is still around and you find you have very little time on your own. When the arrangements are finished and the family have gone home, then that's the time you start to think.

Suddenly the house was silent. I walked around the rooms, remembering the years of our life together. We had been so grateful to move into this house, after living in different lodging houses for almost five years. I opened the bedroom door and looked around, thinking of the laughter we had shared, the hard times, the children we had raised, and the tears we had shed for the babies we had lost. I must have sat on the bed for a good hour or so, reliving our lives, when suddenly it hit me that Joyce wasn't coming back. Not ever, and for the first time since losing her I broke down and sobbed. I stood and walked to the dressing table and took a clean handkerchief from the drawer. On the dressing table stood a music box that Joyce had bought in a charity shop years ago. We had watched a film together in the seventies starring Ali McGraw and Ryan O'Neal, 'The Love Story,' where a young man's heart was broken as he sat and watched his loved one dying of cancer. Joyce had cried all through the film. She also loved the song, 'Where Do I Begin,' by Andy Williams, so she was thrilled when she opened the lid of the music box to find it played that particular song. As I walked away from the dressing table, the music played, just for a second or so. How could it possibly have played without lifting the lid? Had I knocked it when moving away? I didn't think so; I'd already walked away before it played. I don't know how it happened, but I suddenly knew Joyce was in the room beside me.

This was the first time in my life I'd been on my own and I felt incredibly lonely. Little did I know there would be worse to come; I was about to start with an illness that would eventually change my life. Within a year or so of losing Joyce, I realised something was happening to my body and also my mind. Nothing I could tell anyone about. It was hard enough for me to understand, never mind trying to explain these new sensations to someone else. Something was changing; not only on the inside, but on the outside. Each and every task I do is rushed without reason, causing me a great deal of anxiety. On the one hand, I'm slower and my energy seems to have deserted me; yet, my mind is pushing me into daily tasks much more quickly, even when there is no need to hurry. Take for example; on a Tuesday morning regardless of the weather, I'm up and rushing about, ready to join the queue at the post office to collect my pension. I'm not in need of the money . . . not in a way that I have to have it on one particular day, or be stuck in a queue as if the post office is handing out rations. It's just something that has to be done. The gas and electric bills have to be paid on the very day they are due, not a day before or a day after. Rain or shine I still join the dozens of people in the queue.

I hold on to my pension book ready for my turn. Once I'm at the counter, the girls tell me, time and time again.

'You'll be getting mugged one of these days Mr Millar, take your time and put the money in your wallet before going outside. People will have to wait, just like you waited. Stand here and put it away. Pensioners get robbed you know.'

But I still feel rushed and hold the money in my hand until I'm outside.

Returning home, I have the rest of the day in front of me and once more, I'm alone with my thoughts. Eventually I sit down, and try to decide whether I need to see a doctor, and after a great deal of thought, I realise that's not possible. I couldn't explain what's happening to me. What would I say?

'Hello doctor, I'm having trouble sleeping, my finger and my thumb move by themselves, my face has fallen, I'm stiff and I lose my balance. I feel I have to rush but my body won't allow it. I also think I'm depressed, but I don't know how that's supposed to feel. My hand shakes, well one of my hands . . . but I think that's because I drink. I drink because I'm lonely and miss my wife Joyce. Oh . . . and I have a pain in my neck.'

12

The doctor would probably reply, "You are a pain in the neck; take two Paracetamols four times a day . . . Next."

It's hard to explain to anyone how my head feels. I'm being pushed forward by an invisible force, especially when I'm walking and, try as I might, I can't straighten my shoulders back. Being in the army taught me good posture and here I am, suddenly round shouldered, struggling to keep my head up. People have always commented on what a smart man I have been over the years, and I believe good posture has played an important part in those comments. I have always been well groomed and wouldn't dream of stepping out without polished shoes and a tie.

Now when shaving in the mornings, there is a man in the mirror I hardly recognise. My face seems to lack expression, as if my face has dropped down slightly, and my eyes feel different; the only way I can describe it is that I'm staring without blinking. These changes are something I find hard to accept because I've always taken a great pride in my appearance, much to Joyce's amusement.

'Flipping heck, Paddy, we're only walking up to the Co-op for some bread! You've been in that bathroom an hour.'

'Joyce, I haven't been an hour. I've been twenty minutes and I'm almost finished. I'm just getting a shave.'

'How long is that going to take . . . another twenty minutes?'

'Ah go away wid ya. I'll be down in a minute.'

Could these strange sensations I'm feeling be related to depression? I've been lucky enough not to have suffered from depression during my life, and I'm not sure what the symptoms of depression are. I believe it is a feeling of being "fed up" but I'm not quite sure. Joyce used to say she was depressed; but only when her brother, Tom, who she was very close to, died. She used to sit watching the television, but I knew she wasn't really aware of what was happening in the programme. All of a sudden she would burst into tears. Her brother was fifty nine when he died from cancer, and the hard upbringing they had endured together when they lost their father as children, made them very close. From the day Tom died to when Joyce died, she never stopped grieving for him.

I have become aware of a tremor in my left hand, but I assume the reason for the shaking is the amount of alcohol I have started to drink. The tremor is only slight and comes and goes, and as far as I am aware no one else has noticed. It all started with a twitch one day while I was watching television. We all have a twitch now and again, particularly in the eyes when we are over tired, so I thought the feeling would pass. Unfortunately, before the end of the evening the twitch or pulsating was driving me insane. I squeezed my fist together, and then stretched my hand as far as possible. I sat on my hand. I held it tight with my right hand, but still the twitch continued. Finally, I gave up and went to the bathroom for a wash, rubbing my hands with the soap as if I could wash the twitch away. There were days when the pulsating sensation wasn't there, so I began to relax and convince myself it had gone, and was probably something pressing on a nerve. Time went by and I had forgotten about the incident, until I felt that familiar warmth followed by a tiny movement in my finger. It was back.

*

To help pass the time and get away from the quietness of the house during the day, I liked to go to town as much as possible. Even my trip to the post office to pick up my pension was something I looked forward to. The girls who worked there always looked after me, and would even help me choose birthday cards for the family.

'Good morning Patrick, how are you today?' the young girl would ask, as I'm there once again for a card.

'Fine thanks. It's my son's birthday this time.'

She walked over to the racks and showed me the appropriate cards.

'I'll leave you to it; I know you like to take your time reading the verses. If you need me, just give me a call.'

With a family the size of ours I seem to be constantly buying cards, and one day, when I was writing a birthday card out, I was shocked to see how small my handwriting had become. In fact the

14

ink was light coloured, as if there was no pressure at all when I was writing, and I thought I must not have pressed hard enough.

Living a solitary life brings about many new experiences, and I have to admit these days there are times when I am frightened of being on my own. I often think there could be someone downstairs, and sleep with a truncheon at the side of my bed. Tony, my son, brought it back from Spain as a present, and if I had to, I know I would use it. There isn't much point going to bed before midnight as I only sleep for about three hours before waking up again. A lot of the time I stay up late watching the television with the remote control in my hand, flicking from one channel to another, and sometimes I drink more glasses of whisky than I intend to and fall asleep. Suddenly, on one particular evening, I was awoken by a hand on my shoulder shaking me, and I jumped and shouted out. Feeling very startled and confused, I looked up for a second and saw Joyce smiling down on me. 'Joyce . . . Joyce!' I shouted, but she was gone in a flash. This was the second time I had seen her after falling asleep. Was she concerned about my drinking? Was she angry with me? But then, both times she had smiled sympathetically, and I really hoped she wasn't annoyed with me. Not that I would tell anyone I had seen her, mind, they would think I was drunk and had imagined it, but she was there and very real to me.

Later, at the end of the summer season, Tony took me to Blackpool for a weekend. The weather wasn't too good, but we walked on the front for a while, and there was entertainment in the hotel each evening. I think it was about this time that the confusion started to set in. In my room, there were little sachets of milk, coffee, sugar, a kettle and some cups. Tony told me to make a cup of tea whenever I wanted before leaving to go to his own room, but I was still baffled as to what was what. It wasn't as if I had never made a cup of tea, or been in a hotel before, but I was confused with the packets and didn't bother with them, especially after trying to open one. My fingers didn't seem to work properly. I also had trouble with the key to my room; in fact it had taken me a while to open the door. As well as feeling clumsy, I couldn't seem to focus my mind on anything, and I was becoming bewildered and my confidence was dwindling.

It was to be a few months later, the following spring, when I was to stay in a hotel again. This time I had gone to London with Margaret and Geoff, and my great grandson, Nicholas, who was only eight years old. Immediately, Nicholas took control and I was grateful. We were sharing a room together and he was able to use the key card, and he made the tea and coffee. Here I was, being cared for by an eight year old!

*

Margaret had always come through every Friday to help me with my shopping, but now I have started to spend a week out of every month at Margaret's house, which is thirty miles away in West Yorkshire. These visits help to cheer me up. I have my own room there, and have my bag packed and ready to leave two days before going to visit. They run a business, a soft furnishing business, making designer curtains and blinds. Margaret does the sewing and Geoff fits them for the customers. I sit next to her while she sews, reading the paper until later in the day, when I walk down by the canal and sometimes nip into the local pub for a quick drink. I love to stay over at their house and be in company again, and have made quite a few friends just through walking along the canal.

On one of these periodic visits to Margaret's, my secret was about to unfold. I was struggling to put on my coat, getting ready to go out for my walk around the block, and could see her looking at my reflection through the mirror.

'What's the matter with your neck? I saw you flinch when you moved your head just then, and I've also noticed you have a slight stoop, as if your head is pushed forward. Is that because your neck is giving you pain.'

'No, I'm all right.' I lied. 'My neck is just a bit stiff.'

In truth I'm still having pains in my neck, and have had for a while, and my head does feel as if it's being pushed forward.

'It could be the pillows you're using' Margaret said 'you might have too many. I know you like two or three pillows. Or perhaps it could be the weight of your collar pushing your head forward. It's a big heavy coat you're wearing. It might be better to get a lighter one without such a heavy collar. Shall we go shopping tonight at the White Rose shopping centre?'

'That'll be great. I might treat myself to some new trousers. What time will we be going?' I ask her, trying to change the subject away from my neck.

'Well, we'll have something to eat first and then we'll go. It doesn't close while late. I noticed you're having a bit of bother fastening your shoe laces lately. Are your fingers a bit stiff?'

'Yes, it might be a touch of arthritis. I had that once before if you remember.' I lied again.

'Yes, I do remember you wearing some sort of collar around your neck years ago.'

I didn't reply. Why was I lying? Why was I keeping these feelings a secret? I don't know. Probably because I had no idea what was wrong with me. Margaret looked at my shoes.

'You know Dad; they sell men's shoes now that fasten with Velcro. We can look at some today if you like. They'll be a lot easier to fasten than fiddly laces. I wonder if it's arthritis in your neck again as well as your fingers. It needs looking into.'

We arrived at the shopping mall and I chose a nice coat. Margaret was trying to persuade me to buy a hat.

'You need to keep your brain warm you know, you might need it one day.' she laughed. Then on a more serious note she said 'Your hand is shaking a bit. Have you been drinking heavily again?'

Margaret never missed anything. When dropping me off at home one day, she had spotted a bottle of whisky I had hidden behind the settee. She held the half full bottle up in her hand.

'Dad, I wish you would stick to lager. Whisky is not good for you, it rots the liver. Me mam will be turning in her grave. She hated you drinking large amounts of alcohol. In fact, she hated you drinking at all after your heart attack and bypass.'

I stood there with my head down, feeling ashamed of myself and I promised to give up drinking whisky. We paid for the hat, and I told Margaret I hadn't bought any more whisky since the day she found the bottle. I told her I only had a couple of cans a night.

'Anyway, come on, we'll have a coffee' she said, plonking the hat on my head, 'I believe you, thousands wouldn't, as me mam used to say.'

A few days later it was time to pack my bags and go home, and I was already looking forward to my next visit to their house. The week had just flown by.

As usual, I returned from Margaret's on a Sunday, calling at the supermarket first for my groceries. She always helps me put my shopping away and check upstairs to make sure everything is all right in the house before leaving. There was always that same sad look on her face when she waved goodbye to me and drove off into the night. Still, my son Tony comes and spends a couple of hours with me on Sunday evenings, and I look forward to our chats. He's always optimistic with me and tries his best to help me carry on without Joyce. But even he has seen the changes in me. Once, near to Christmas, he asked me when I was going to put the tree up.

'I'm not putting one up this year,' I said in a low, sorry for myself voice. 'There's no point. I'm going to Margaret's for Christmas. Anyway, I can't see the point of putting decorations up when you're on your own.'

'Dad there's every point. You have a family and grandchildren here, and they may want to come to see you at some time over Christmas. You always used to put the decorations up early when me mam was alive. You both loved to trim up, and the house was always very Christmassy . . . even if you just put up the tree and Christmas cards, it's better than having no decorations at all.'

Tony looked at me and went quiet for a few seconds and his face softened.

'You need to start living again Dad. It's been hard for us all. We all miss me mam, but life goes on. She wouldn't want you to give up. She looked after you when you had your heart attack and by-pass operation, and she made herself ill with worry over you. You can't give in Dad.'

I tried to get a word in, but couldn't, and I knew he was right in what he was saying.

'You have a good life when you look at it really. You're always tripping off somewhere with Margaret and Geoff, and you enjoy going to stay there. You meet up with Teresa twice during the week for a meal in town, Kev calls in now and again, and I still can't understand why you stopped going to the club with your neighbour, Shaun . . . you used to enjoy it. You also enjoyed going to Patricks on a Saturday night. You liked Saturday nights there.'

I didn't want to tell Tony I'd started to drink whisky in the club, and sometimes turned a bit argumentative. We used to take it in turns to buy rounds of drinks, and Shaun had told his brothers not to buy me whisky anymore. He could see how it was changing my personality. I was once told to 'shhh' when they were playing bingo and I lost my temper. I had become so bitter and angry, and this was something no-one had ever seen in me, including myself. So I made the excuse to Tony that it was a bit boring when they played bingo.

'Well you could go into the taproom while it's over like the others do. Margaret comes over to take you shopping when you're at home, as well as you staying there every month. She has a business to run, but puts herself out to look after you Dad. Your life couldn't be better under the circumstances.'

I knew my depression was bringing him down, and I was also making him feel depressed, but I couldn't help myself. I also knew I was always feeling sorry for myself, when once I had always had a positive and happy outlook on life. I used to love company and taking part in conversations, but now I have no interest in anything apart from drinking. On top of that, something else was happening to me. I was beginning to repeat myself. I was often told I had said something twice, but I couldn't remember doing it. This started to

19

make me very wary of saying anything in case I had already said it. After a while, people stopped telling me I was repeating myself, and I assumed they were letting me believe they had heard it for the first time.

What is happening to me? Will somebody please tell me?

Chapter Three

Diagnosis

(2003)

The phone rang and I quickly grabbed hold of it and said 'Hello.'

Margaret's voice was on the other end of the line.

'Were you sitting on the phone again Dad.' she laughed.

'Erm, no, I was just passing as it rang.'

We both laughed as she knew that wasn't true, the telephone couldn't be any nearer to me. Sometimes I would grab the phone so fast, that it would fall to the floor and cut me off.

'Anyway Dad, I know you've only just got home, but do you fancy coming over here seeing as its Easter, we can go to the coast if you like? I know it's raining but we might as well go somewhere instead of sitting in all weekend. What do you think?'

'That'll be great. I'll bring my new coat, its waterproof.'

'What's the best day to pick you up? Shall we say Thursday?'

'Oh Thursday will be grand. I won't be doing anything then.'

Margaret laughed. 'Dad, no matter what day I suggest you come over here, you always say that, just as if you had a full diary.' We both laughed again and she said she would see me on Friday.

'Friday. . .' I shouted, 'I thought you said Thursday.'

'Just testing; see you Thursday Dad.'

Thursday arrived, and I went through the house making sure everything was in order. Plugs were unplugged and the two back doors locked and bolted. I made myself another cup of tea and poured the rest of the milk down the sink. I'd forgotten to do this once and the milk had gone off, leaving a bad smell in the house. When everything was in order I sat on the chair nearest to the front door with my bags ready. Because of her business, it wasn't possible for Margaret to state a time, other than sometime in the morning, so I sat and waited for her. When she came through the door, I immediately jumped up and picked up my bags.

She smiled when she saw me. 'Have you been sitting there all morning with those bags in your hand?'

'No' I laughed, because she knew I had.

During the car journey, whilst driving, she was looking at my hand.

'Dad, I'm not happy about the way your hand is shaking. I thought it must be with you drinking too much, but surely that would affect both your hands, not just one? I think you should see a doctor. In fact, I might take you to see my doctor because your doctor is useless. Look how he was with me mam, and how he treated you for sciatica when really you had an impacted bowel. You told him you were badly constipated and still he gave you tablets that clearly stated they could make you constipated. I've seen you trying to hide the shaking from me. It might not be anything sinister, but we need to know. By the way, another thing I've noticed, you don't seem to swing your arms as much when walking. You seem very rigid. You were always a fast walker, now you walk much more slowly.'

I tried to tuck my hand out of the way. I'd noticed myself how slower my steps were, but hadn't really thought about whether my arms moved.

I hoped Margaret would forget about taking me to see her doctor, but I was wrong. A few days later we went to see her GP and Margaret introduced me to the doctor.

'This is my dad, Patrick. I know it might be nothing to worry about, but for a while now there seems to have been a bit of a tremor in his hand. He also has a stiff neck that pushes his head forward, and I wondered if he was developing symptoms of Parkinson's disease. I don't know anything about Parkinson's other than their hands shake, so I've brought him to this surgery because he stays with us quite a lot. In fact he almost lives with us now.'

The doctor stood up and shook my hand.

'Hello Patrick. There are all kinds of different things which can cause our hands to shake. Let's have a look at you, shall we.'

I always find it strange that the British often say 'we' and not 'I'. The doctor asked me to take off my coat and shirt to get a good look at my neck. He listened to my chest and back with a stethoscope, and I was asked to walk across the room and back again. Sitting down, he wrote a few notes before he told me I could put my shirt back on. This took me a few moments as recently I was having trouble fastening buttons, almost as if my hands were too big. I was sure that buttons were bigger than the button holes these days. I heard the doctor say something to Margaret as I struggled to dress, but the only bit I clearly overheard from the conversation was that I needed to see my own GP.

'What's Parkinson's disease?' I asked on our drive home.

'I'm not really sure myself, other than you have a shaky hand and stiff neck, but whatever it is, we'll get to the bottom of it. I'm sure there's help for it. That's if it *is* Parkinson's disease, we don't know yet. You heard what the doctor said; there could be a number of reasons for your hand shaking.'

Margaret arranged an appointment with my own GP for when I went home. I hadn't told her that I had missed a hospital appointment about my hernia, and I was reluctant to go in case the doctor said something to me about it. I mentioned this to Margaret on the morning we were driving to the surgery.

'I couldn't find the letter anywhere, yer mam always did that sort of thing. I'm dreading going, the doctor will be annoyed with me.'

23

'Dad, those days are gone when we used to put doctors on a high pedestal. They do a wonderful job, but they are only human beings, just like the rest of us. I can't believe you are so worried about going to see the doctor. Surely, he won't yell at you for losing a letter?'

My name was called. It was the lady doctor, and as usual she didn't look up from her desk when we entered the room. That was how she always was and her husband was just the same. Margaret let me sit down before saying to her.

'I've been asked by my doctor to bring Dad in for a check up as he has a tremor in his hand . . .'

The doctor ignored her and looked at me.

'Why did you miss your hospital appointment for your Hernia?'

'Erm, I lost the letter . . .'

Margaret quickly butted in as I sat there looking down at the floor.

'His memory isn't very good these days and he couldn't remember where he put the letter.'

The doctor kept her head down, looking at the notes on her desk. She hadn't even looked at Margaret. She totally ignored her. After reading something from the notes, the doctor muttered.

'Well that's to be expected with Parkinson's disease. I'll make an appointment for you to see the Parkinson's specialist, and another appointment for your Hernia. Try not to lose this appointment letter.'

That was it; she was done with me. I was dismissed. We were silent almost all the way home, until Margaret spoke.

'Dad, you really need to change your doctor. That was ridiculous; who does she think she is? If it wasn't for you having to see her again on your own, I would have had plenty to say to her. I can't believe you put up with that crap from her. She was so rude and ignorant. Doctors are not like that. In all my life, I've never known a doctor like yours; our doctor even shook your hand when

24

I introduced you. Most doctors do these days, or at least they acknowledge you. No wonder me mam dreaded going to that surgery. She should have had home visits the state she was in, not be trailing up that hill just weeks before she died, all because the doctor wouldn't come out to see her. Jesus Christ, what a way to deliver the news to someone they have Parkinson's disease.'

'But how did she know I have Parkinson's disease? She didn't examine me.'

'She'll have had a letter from my GP, and anyway, they only suspect its Parkinson's disease Dad. You haven't seen the specialist yet.'

I hoped it wasn't. It was true about my memory. I had become very forgetful lately. What really surprised me was that Margaret had noticed, although she never said anything. But then again, did she say something and I had forgotten. I thought about what Margaret had said about the doctor.

'At least it wasn't her husband. He has worse manners than she has,' I said bitterly, 'and he was awful to yer mam. He was always very abrupt with her. She could hardly walk during those last few weeks before she was admitted to hospital. I know no-one knew at the time she had cancer, but the doctor made her out to be paranoid each time she went to the surgery. He even told her a few months earlier that it wasn't cancer, saying "it isn't cancer if that's what you're thinking." He used to insist she went to the surgery so he could examine her better, even though he knew we didn't have a car and it was a long walk from our house.'

'I know Dad. It's hard to believe she was only diagnosed about three or four weeks before she died. By that time the cancer had spread to her bones and everywhere. It breaks my heart to think how much she must have suffered those last few months at home.'

'She certainly did suffer. She used to go into the back bedroom when she thought I was sleeping. I would follow her in there to find her sitting on the bed, her arms wrapped tightly around her body, rocking to and fro with pain. I feel so guilty now for not pursuing it further. I should have insisted she was referred to a specialist.'

Margaret was very angry with my GP and said firmly. 'Well, I did try to get you both in at the doctors down the road from your house. I got you the forms and everything. They even accepted you both, but me mam changed her mind at the last minute.'

'I know. Yer mam didn't like change, I wish we had taken your advice and changed doctors now.'

'Still, it's not too late for you, you know. I'm not sure I can sit there and let that woman speak to you in that way ever again.'

Margaret had a coffee before setting off home. She was still fuming with the doctor and the way she spoke to me. 'She didn't explain anything to us, and as for losing a letter, how dare she speak to you like a child? God, I wish I'd said something. But then you have to see her when I'm not with you. It's high time you changed doctors Dad.'

When I was on my own I started to think about what the doctor had said. Parkinson's . . . Disease. . . Memory loss . . . What was Parkinson's disease? Whatever it was, it had something to do with memory loss. Oh God! What was that disease me auld mate had? He didn't even remember his wife. He couldn't remember anything. We went to see him and he didn't even know his friends, he looked right through us. Alzheimer's or something, that's what it must be. I must have Alzheimer's.

'Oh my God, please, not that'.

Things were beginning to make sense. The pain in my legs, the cramp in my feet, the stiffness in my neck, the shaking, and not being able to sleep were just some of the problems my body was battling with. Now I was losing my memory. I was sure that was the first sign of Alzheimer's or dementia.

The next time I saw Margaret, she said she'd noticed a change in me. She probably had. I felt different. It didn't matter how much she tried to reassure me it wasn't Alzheimer's or Dementia, I wasn't convinced. To make matters worse, my head aches were much worse and the doctor was referring me for a brain scan. I was worried about the very thought of that, and the outcome of it.

'Dad, the scan has nothing to do with Parkinson's or any other disease. It's because you are having a lot of headaches. It's probably with drinking. You hadn't had a drink for years before me mam died. Now your body must be wondering what the hell you're doing to it. The scan doesn't hurt at all, nothing touches you. It's only like an x-ray.'

Margaret was right; I didn't even have to take my clothes off. I just lay down on a table with my head under a machine that spun round. The machine looked to me as if it had come out of a Science Fiction film. Shortly afterwards, I was informed that an arthritic nerve was the cause of my headaches.

I was told to take two paracetamol tablets, four times a day.

A month went by and I had an appointment letter for the Parkinson's clinic. I phoned   Margaret up straight away to tell her.

'A letter has come this morning for a hospital appointment and it's for a week on Monday, will you be coming with me?' I asked, hoping she would say yes.

'What time is it for?'

'The appointment is for nine in the morning.' I replied and it went a little quiet before she answered.

'That means I'll have to set off from here at seven thirty. It'll be busy at that time.' Another pause and then, 'Okay. I'll see you get there and then you can come back here with me if you want. We'll have to get straight back, I have some curtains to finish off and they're booked to be fitted.'

As soon as I had put the phone back on the hook I was off to pack my bag, even though it was over a week away. If I could, I would have taken two stairs at a time. I settled for one step, pulling on the hand rail to get up there more quickly.

On the day of the appointment, we finally found the clinic. It seemed a long walk from the other part of the hospital. I had to be weighed and then pee into a plastic tub. We waited over an hour before seeing the consultant, and apparently, there is no test as such for Parkinson's. The consultant asked me to walk up and down the tiny room. He asked me to lift my arms up in the air, before asking me to sit down. Holding my wrists, he moved my hands up and down as if to shake them. The consultant seemed to be looking at my face quite a lot and later, I was told they look for facial expressions, *or lack of them.* Finally he asked for background information about my health and how I was feeling at the time.

Writing out a prescription for some medication, I was given another appointment for six months' time. That was that, finished, the end of the appointment which I had waited all those months for. I was dismissed for the second time without any explanation. I wasn't given any information as to what Parkinson's disease was. It wasn't even a Parkinson's clinic; all the brochures and leaflets were for stroke patients. We had to wait a further twenty minutes in the pharmacy for my new medication until finally; we were on our way home.

*

It's been quite a few weeks since my appointment with the Parkinson's specialist. Nothing much else seems to have changed, except by this time my arm is shaking as well as my hand. In the evenings when I am on my own, I get very angry and hit my hand quite hard leaving a big bruise. I find that when I'm stressed or angry, my hand shakes more and I feel like chopping it off.

When I saw the specialist, he prescribed me a tablet called Sinemet, which is supposed to stop all the shaking. Of course, I still need to take all of my heart tablets. Each and every day I take my daily tablets out of a little container which has the days of the week written on the lid. Margaret bought it and showed me how to fill it up for the week, but I still struggle. Joyce had always seen to my heart medication. Margaret rings at 8:00am to make sure I have taken the first lot, and to make sure I remember to take the ones at lunch time. At tea time she rings again.

Had I already put that one in? Which one do I need to take in the afternoon?

Had it not been for the fact that I was at my son Patrick's house one night, I probably wouldn't be here now. He was concerned when I first arrived and asked if I had been drinking, which I hadn't. He said my speech was slurred and my eyes looked a little strange, and within a short time of arriving there, I fell asleep; which was totally out of character for me at the time. Patrick and his friend took me to the casualty department at our local hospital, but not before calling home to pick up my medication. Somehow, I had got mixed up with my tablets; I was accidently overdosing and had been doing so for a few days or possibly longer. I was very nervous after that particular incident, and went from overdosing to missing them completely. I was confused beyond belief. Sometimes the colour of the tablets changed. I would get used to a certain colour, and the following month the colour of the tablets would be different. Even the shape of tablets altered time and time again, and sometimes I would have two identical looking tablets. Getting into a packet was hard enough, especially the blister packs. The bloody pills would end up falling on the floor and disappear. And the dreaded child proof lids still frustrate me as I struggle to open them. It would be so much easier if the tablets stayed the same shape and colour each month. Do the manufacturers of bottles and blister packs ever give a thought to the elderly?

As winter sets in, the curtains are not drawn until the very last drop of light fades, and then the lamps are switched on. These very lamps that made the house look like a cosy home, now give no sense of cosiness. I am very frightened of this disease that is invading my body, particularly when I am alone. Some evenings I suddenly feel very emotional and angry at Joyce for leaving me. I scream at her photograph as if she is in the room.

'Joyce, why did you leave me? Why did you have to go? What have I got left now? Oh Joyce I miss you.'

29

Throwing the television remote control across the room, I break down and cry. Am I changing into a monster? I'm so scared of living a life with this illness and being without Joyce. I know I would have been able to cope if she was with me. Fifty years we had together. She has taken a part of me with her and left the other bit behind. I feel so weepy all the time. What is happening to me?

This feeling of dread and sadness fills every part of my body and mind. I am going deeper into despair. My family tries to reassure me I don't have Alzheimer's or Dementia, but I'm forever repeating myself. I can tell by the look on their faces. Even I am aware that I must have said it before. I'm also having nightmares where something is eating my mind away, and I dream of Joyce as if she is alive. I talk to her in my dreams and see her smiling face, but when I awake she is gone, leaving me lonelier than ever. Some nights I lay awake on my bed staring at the ceiling, trying to make sense of it all. Thinking of the questions I would ask if I was given the chance.

Is Parkinson's disease the cause of everything that's happening to me now?

Does it run in families?

Will my children get it?

How did I get it?

Is it curable?

Will it shorten my life? Jaysus! Am I going to die?

Is it because of drinking so much in my younger years?

Is it because I was always banging my head when I worked on the building sites?

Who will help me with the answers to these questions?

Margaret is concerned about me feeling down, and tells me I am depressed and suffering from grief. She thinks depression may be a symptom of Parkinson's and arranges for me to see my doctor who gives me antidepressants, something called Prozac. But of course the doctor didn't give me an explanation as to why I feel the way I do. I feel in my heart it is more than grief. After Margaret left for home, I put the tablets down the toilet. I had heard of Prozac . . . once you were on them you couldn't come off them, and some people go on to take even stronger drugs. There are days when I won't take my Parkinson's medication, just for the defiance of it all. I believe they are the cause of my awful nightmares, and I hate the fact that I have to take so many pills. I am turning into a very bitter man.

WHAT IS PARKINSON'S DISEASE? They have given me the title of something incurable, without giving me an explanation of what is to happen as the disease progresses.

Finally, I received another appointment to see the specialist about my hernia. It was my own fault for losing the first letter in the first place, and I had waited three months for the appointment. In the meantime, a letter came from my doctor informing me I was due for a routine blood test, for my Cholesterol levels at the hospital. I phoned Margaret to ask if she would come with me, and I gave her the details and the date.

'Dad, you mentioned the letter says you can't have anything to eat or drink from 9:00pm the night before, and until after the blood test. You have to stick to that you know. This means no beer after nine and no tea in the morning.'

'Okay, I won't forget.'

She came to take me to the hospital, but on the way there I told her I had drunk a cup of tea. Margaret was not happy with me.

'They won't do the blood test now, I've come thirty miles for nothing and I'm up to my eyes in work. I can't believe you Dad.'

'I won't tell them, they don't need to know.'

'They tell you not to eat or drink for a reason.'

When we arrived at the hospital they asked if I had had anything to eat or drink, besides water for my tablets. Margaret told them I had drunk a small cup of tea and they refused to do the blood test, and arranged another appointment.

To make matters worse, after seeing the specialist about my hernia and being told I needed surgery, there were problems on the day of the operation. I was all packed and prepared when Margaret arrived to take me to the hospital. We were in a waiting room for five hours only to be told there were no beds available, and I was asked if I could I come back the following day. Margaret came to take me to the hospital for the second time, and once more we were told the same thing, there were no beds. This was after waiting four hours in a small room. Margaret was not happy.

'Well' she said to the ward sister, who had delivered the news, 'I tell you what, you find him a bed because I'm leaving him here if you don't. You can sort it out. I'm not coming thirty miles to bring him here for a third time. My dad has suffered from this condition for years and he has Parkinson's and heart disease. He does not need this kind of stress at his age.'

Later, Margaret told me she would never have left me there on my own, but she was angry because they had turned down her request to phone her when they had a bed for me. She said it wasn't the fact that she'd come a long way, it was the hours we had spent in the waiting room only to be told there wasn't a bed for the second time. After waiting for a further five hours a bed was found for me at seven in the evening, and I was operated on the following morning. When I left the hospital I went to Margaret's while I recovered.

*

It was at this time when she decided to come out of the shop and work from home, and I was amazed to see how much the sewing had taken over the house. There was fabric just about everywhere and in every room. Curtains were hung all around my bedroom walls, waiting to be packed, and my bed had to be cleared of half-finished curtains before I could sleep in it. The room where Margaret worked from was so crowded with sewing products, machines and fabric that she seemed to disappear amid it all. Threads of cotton stuck to our shoes and left a trail of thread all over the house. The lovely home they once had was now like a sewing factory. After our evening meal we discussed how things

32

couldn't carry on as they were, and that they had decided to look for bigger premises.

'We thought we could rent a bigger house to start with, rather than buy, and in the near future we can look at buying a house nearer to you, and perhaps build an extension to use as a workroom. But for now, we need a bigger house quickly.'

Everything happened very fast, and after a few weeks of searching for the right place, they finally found the ideal house. It had five good sized bedrooms, three upstairs and two downstairs, more than enough rooms for a large cutting table and three industrial sewing machines. The back of the house overlooked the river Aire, where there were fantastic views over Ilkley moor, but, although we had the wonderful scenery, the end of the garden was a sheer drop of about fifty feet into bushes, trees and nettles. This was a concern for all of us, as Margaret had four grandchildren, my great grandchildren. Through the large window, you could see deer running around the woodlands and herons standing tall in the shallow parts of the river, ready to dip their heads down and swoop up with a fish. The back garden was so peaceful; it was almost like being away from civilisation.

At the front of the house there was a large porch and a patio, which was petitioned off from the rest of the garden. A secret garden, as Margaret called it. Within a short time, Geoff had made a pond in-between the flag stones, and it was great on a summers evening, watching the fish swimming around and hearing the birds chirping away. I was spending more and more time at Margaret and Geoff's, and I was less troubled about my condition. Perhaps it was because they made sure I was taking my medication regularly, and eating properly that had brought about this stabilisation of my symptoms. Life really was good that summer. I seemed to be holding my own with Parkinson's disease, and I am glad to say that nothing much had changed since I was diagnosed. The tablets seemed to help with my stiffness and shaking, and I believed I was not repeating myself as much, at least no one had said anything for a long time.

My bedroom at Margaret's new home was upstairs on a long corridor, and at the far end of the corridor, a big bedroom door faced you as you walked towards it. The bathroom was on the left hand side and the two other rooms, including mine, were further down on the right hand side. The strange thing about the bedroom at the end of the corridor, was that it had two bolts on the outside of the door, and inside the room it had its own sink and bathroom cabinet. I couldn't help but wonder why there were locks on the outside of the door.

Was someone mad locked up there?

I really didn't like walking down the corridor during the night, especially as I was the only one who slept upstairs, unless the grandchildren stayed over. So I always used the downstairs bathroom before I went to bed, but of course I still had to go to the bathroom again during the night. When I did go, I would turn on the light, and walk with my head down towards the bolted bedroom door that faced me. Even entering the upstairs bathroom itself was eerie, because it had another door inside that led to a storage room. This inner door didn't close properly, and left a gap through which I could just make out shapes on the other side. There I would stand and pee, keeping my face to the front, whistling a tune, half expecting someone to jump out and shout '*Boo*'.

Margaret and Geoff's bedroom was downstairs, and the other bedroom next to theirs was used as a cutting room, and had a table that almost filled the whole room. The lounge, where we all sat on an evening watching the television, was very big with window seats in the bay and, as Margaret said after trying different ways of arranging the furniture, it was too big to make cosy. She did her sewing at the back of the house in another large room which had plenty of light and overlooked the river. There seemed to be rooms everywhere, including a large hall which led out onto the porch. It was the kind of house that could be used in a horror movie, or an Agatha Christie crime drama.

When I lay in my bed, I could hear creaks and groans from the house cooling down, and sometimes it sounded like footsteps creeping towards my room. I wished Margaret and Geoff's room was upstairs, but the only double room upstairs was the one down the corridor with the bolted door, and Margaret didn't like that room! I always tried getting off to sleep before Geoff turned out the hall light downstairs. I had my bedside light if I needed it, but the rest of the house was in complete darkness. Eventually, I would drift off into a deep sleep.

I leave my bedroom to go to the toilet at the end of the corridor, the lights are dim, but I can see. On my way back, I hear a man's voice behind me, coming from the room with locks and bolts. I try to run but my body is in slow motion and I feel as if I'm walking without moving. I open my mouth to shout for help, but my face is paralysed and I struggle to breathe. I'm dying. I thrash around fighting for air. Suddenly I feel the warmth of someone's hand on my shoulder, followed by a loud crash.

I was awake, woken by the crash. The clock from the side of my bed was on the floor along with the lamp. I must have knocked them off the table when I was thrashing about. I was wet through from sweat and had tightness in my chest. Was I about to have a heart attack? Whose hand did I feel on my shoulder? Was it Joyce?

I told Margaret about my dream and she could see I was still pretty shaken by it. She handed me a cup of tea and as usual had a logical explanation.

'It's probably because you said the corridor put you in mind of that horror film . . . oh! What's its name now? You know Dad, Jack Nicholson was in it. It was snowing and he had an axe . . . '

'The Shining' I said quietly.

'Yeah that's the one, The Shining. Some of the medication you take can cause sweating. Of course, you might have had a touch of Angina all the same. If you have any more chest pains or tightness, let me know and I'll take you to our doctors to get a check-up.'

'I'm all right now, but I've been feeling really strange for a while and my headaches have got worse. I feel light headed and once or twice I felt as though I was going to faint. Sometimes when I stand up it's like a dark curtain coming down over my eyes.'

'It's probably your blood pressure lowering. It might be an idea to stand up more slowly Dad.'

'I usually do, but I feel weak and tired all the time, and have a strange sensation of being out of my body.'

Margaret looked concerned. 'I think we ought to take a visit to the doctors. It could be the medication.'

Is this another symptom of Parkinson's or the effects of the medication? It seems to get rid of poison, you have to take poison.

*

Summer had its ups and downs, but in general the time passed without too many problems. Once autumn arrived, I was spending my time living between my house and Margaret's, which happened to be eerily quiet on those dark evenings. At the back of the building, there were no street lamps, just sheer darkness and trees swaying in the wind, looking like shadows moving in the night. Being such a big house meant there were lots of light bulbs and if one bulb blew, all the lights would go out, including the ones on the outside of the house. The lights seemed to be constantly blowing a fuse and Geoff thought there must be an electrical fault as the bulbs didn't last as long as they should. To make matters worse, the switch box was down in the cellar, which was as large as the ground floor of the house, and also had several rooms.

I carried on as normal spending some of the time in my own house, but I hadn't been home for more than a week when Margaret rang.

'Hello Dad, how are you? Do you fancy coming back here; it's lonely with Geoff being out all day. I miss your company, as well as someone to keep me going with cups of tea while I work.' She laughed; 'Guess what, I've joined a Buddhist group down in Saltaire. It's somewhere to go for a change. I needed to get out of the house, and it was all I could find when I went to the library to see if there were any courses nearby which might interest me.'

The day after she phoned, she picked me up and I was back again. Margaret went to her first Buddha meeting, telling us all about the meditation when she came home. She went to quite a few of their meetings, and one day I was shocked to find she had invited a couple of Buddhist monks over to the house. One looked to be at least six feet four inches tall, with a wide grin which spread from ear to ear. His hair had been shaved off, and he was dressed in a long orange gown that made him appear to tower, even more so, above everyone else.

After a while however, Margaret decided that Buddhism was boring and wasn't for her after all. The whole Buddhist class had gone out for a meal, and she was shocked to see that they had all ordered water, when she had ordered a bottle of wine. Off she went to the library again to find something else and came back with an armful of books on hypnotherapy.

'There's a course coming up in Selby and it's the first weekend of every month. It lasts for a year, so it's very expensive, but you can pay monthly.'

At the beginning of the following month, she came home after the first session, wanting to practice it on anyone that would let her, eager to show her new talent off.

'I'll have a go on you, Dad, to see if I can stop your hand shaking.'

I had been feeling dizzy and sick earlier in the morning, and still felt a little light headed, but didn't say anything about it. I also had a bad headache. She sat me in a recliner chair and started to speak in a very low voice, just enough for me to hear her. I became really relaxed listening to the sound of her voice and the soft music in the background, and I had a feeling of floating away. I can't remember anything else other than Margaret shouting my name. When I open my eyes I was shocked to see two ambulance men standing at the side of me, trying to talk to me. I had passed out. Luckily, when Margaret rang for an ambulance, there was one only a few yards from the house, which was on its way back to the depot. After hearing about my past medical history they decided to take me to Leeds hospital. Margaret was distraught; believing she was the one who had caused me to pass out, but the paramedics assured her it was nothing to do with hypnosis. On the way to the hospital, I was asked by the paramedic if I had any pain. I slowly put my hand on my heart and nodded my head. When we arrived, I was rushed into a side ward because they assumed I could be having a heart attack, especially when Margaret told them about the night when I woke up wet through from sweating, and had tightness in my chest.

I was taken into a side room, and it wasn't very long before the doctor came to see me. After a quick examination and questions, he arranged for blood tests and x-rays to be taken. The doctor came back to the room an hour later holding an x ray in his hand and by the serious look on his face I feared he was going to tell me I had suffered a heart attack.

'Mr Millar, do you drink much alcohol?'

'I only drink a couple of lagers a night.' I said very quietly to the doctor, but Margaret had a look of disbelief on her face, and was shocked to hear me tell such a lie. She looked at me and turned to the doctor.

'Yes he does. He drinks far too much . . . whisky as well. He didn't drink over the past thirty years or so . . . only very occasionally, and in small amounts, but he seems to have turned to alcohol now he lives on his own . . . more so since he was diagnosed with Parkinson's disease. My mother died a few years ago and he isn't eating properly when he's on his own at home. I don't think he can be bothered. Often, when I go to pick him up from home, the food we bought the previous week can still be in the fridge. He has a meal when he goes into town with my sister, and when he's staying with us he eats very well, but he does drink quite a lot of alcohol when he's on his own. On top of that, sometimes he doesn't take his medication for Parkinson's disease because he gets confused with the dosage. It's as if he's lost the will to live.'

The doctor listened with interest as she told him about my drinking, and the fact that I didn't look after myself properly because I was suffering from grief. The doctor looked down at me and I was waiting to be told off.

'Mr Millar, your liver is not looking good at the moment, and if you carry on drinking at this level, you will die. You are also suffering from Hypoglycaemia, which is why you probably passed out, and may also be the cause of the sweating, headaches and feeling tired. You are, in addition, malnourished from going without food for long periods of time, and drinking too much alcohol. This is why you may feel dizzy and unsteady. However, the good news is that your heart is fine, but we will be keeping you in for a while, just to be on the safe side and to do some more tests.'

It wasn't the first time I had passed out since Joyce had died, and each time the medics arrived I was asked if I had any pain, and I would nod my head and hold my chest. I didn't have a pain in my chest . . . I never had, not since I had a bypass. But I had no idea what was happening to me, and assumed it must be my heart.

I was given bottles of Lucozade to drink and taken to a ward, where I stayed for a week. The doctor did some more tests and said physically I was all right, but he thought I was suffering from depression. I started to cry at that point, which was totally out of character for me. The doctor was very sympathetic and understanding.

'A lot of people suffer from depression after the loss of a loved one, but drinking alcohol in excess only makes the depression worse. Plus, the medication you take for Parkinson's disease can cause dizziness and fainting, so it's important that you eat regularly to stop your blood sugar from going up and down. This is another reason to cut down on drink. You can still drink alcohol Mr Millar, but just make sure it's at a safe level, and try not to go too long without food when you are on your own.'

The doctor suggested I try some antidepressants for a while, and explained they are not addictive as some people believe. He told me the tablets are to help people get over a bad time in their life.

'Sometimes people get depressed when they have Parkinson's disease, and many patients have found antidepressants to be a great help.'

The doctor explained I may only need them for a short time, before gradually coming off them once I felt well enough to do so. I decided to take the tablets this time and make sure that I ate my meals, and cut down on my drinking.

When I was discharged from the hospital I spent a week with Margaret and Geoff, recuperating until I went home. I was feeling pretty glum when I returned to my house after staying there and being spoilt. A week later the phone rang.

'Hiya dad, me and Geoff have been talking, I'm not happy living at this house. It's too isolated for me to be on my own all the time, and the rent is unbelievably high. Which means we're back to working hard to pay the overheads again. We have decided to look for a house to buy with a bedroom for you to use, then you can live with us permanently . . . that's if you want to. We can't stand back and let you kill yourself, and we really don't mind you living with us, you more or less live with us now anyway . . . but don't be packing yet, it'll be a while,' she laughed.

While Geoff was at work, Margaret and I went looking at houses that were on the market. We drove around for hours looking for a house in the right area. The ones that were affordable weren't big enough for her to do her sewing, and allow me to live there as well. They needed at least a three bed roomed house, so they also had enough room for the grandchildren to stay over in the holidays, and enough land on which to build an extension to convert into a workroom. Geoff was hoping they would be able to buy a house in West Yorkshire so he could travel to work easily, as he fitted curtains and blinds for other firms as well as for Margaret. Unfortunately, if the house we looked at was big enough, then the area wasn't suitable, and vice versa.

After weeks of disappointment, I suggested they moved in with me with a view to buying the house. I live in a large three bed roomed house with huge gardens to the front, back and side. There was plenty of room for extensions and is situated in a good area with a large open field at the back and a green to the front, and Margaret could use the biggest bedroom for sewing until the extension was built. Although my house was not in West

40

Yorkshire, it was still near enough for Geoff to travel to work as it's quite close to the motorway. They liked the idea, and agreed it was a good solution to all the problems of working and taking care of me.

However, before moving into the house, Geoff wanted to make some alterations. It was decided that I live with Margaret in Cottingley, and Geoff move into my house to fit a new bathroom and do a bit of redecorating. Being in the house without anyone else to think about, meant he could get more work done in the evenings. It also meant he didn't have to worry about turning the water off for long periods of time while he did the plumbing.

Back at Cottingley, the house seemed really quiet without Geoff. Margaret slept in the downstairs bedroom and I stayed upstairs in my room. I know she was anxious with Geoff not being at home, because she slept with the light on in the hall. One evening while watching the television in the lounge, we were startled by a noise in the kitchen. The floorboards creaked as if someone was walking towards us. I grabbed the nearest thing to me, which was a heavy candlestick lamp, and Margaret laughed as I held it in my hand without unplugging it. Whispering, she asked if I intended electrocuting the intruder. I laughed and she told me to shush. We listened very quietly and I couldn't help but think about the 'Cluedo' board game.

Mr Millar murdered in the kitchen with a candlestick.

I was about to say this to Margaret when suddenly we were plunged into total blackness as all the lights went out. Luckily, Margaret was always burning candles so there were plenty to hand, although we had to fumble about for the matches . . . which were not at hand. Because Bonny, our dog, wasn't barking, Margaret whispered to me that there couldn't be anyone in the house, still, I didn't like the idea of her going down into the cellar in the dark to flick the switch back up. I stood at the top of the stairs holding a candle in one hand and the candlestick lamp in the other, while she walked down to the cellar with a torch she had found on a shelf at the top of the stairs. She switched the lights back on and ran back to the top, two stairs at a time. I had insisted on going down to put the switch back up myself, but she said I would end up breaking my neck on the concrete stairs. The outside lights still wouldn't work. It was very dark outside and I didn't like the worried look Margaret had on her face.

'I hope it's not druggies Dad. They might have tried to cut the electric wire or something.'

'But the inside lights work now. It must be another fuse.'

'Yeah, I suppose so, but if its drug dealers, they might think we're rich living in a house this size, and we're not that far from the City centre where there are a lot of drug dealers.'

'Should we ring Geoff?'

'I don't know Dad, what if we have him coming all this way just because of a fuse. Bonny seems all right, and she can hear if someone comes to the house long before we even hear them. I think we'll be all right. It might have been the floorboards creaking.'

The rest of the evening we watched television while watching Bonny's face, and every time she moved we stiffened up listening for noises. Most of the time she only stretched out and yawned, but occasionally she would lift her head up as if she had heard a sound, before looking at the pair of us staring down at her. Any other time it would have been funny, Bonny looking at us and us looking at her. She must have been puzzled that night wondering why we were so interested in her.

We eventually went to bed, leaving all the lights on. I just hoped they didn't blow a fuse again, because even with the lights on, I had to face the walk down the corridor to the bathroom. I didn't relish the thought of walking down the corridor with a candle in my hand . . . not in this house. The corridor really did put me in mind of the film 'The Shining' and I half expected Jack Nicholson to come running out with an axe in his hand shouting 'Honey I'm home' before slicing me in two. From day one I believed someone was in the bolted room and it gave me the creeps. I thought of how funny Joyce would have found the fact that I was frightened of a room at the end of a corridor.

42

Thankfully, after three weeks Geoff had finished decorating the rooms and had put a new bathroom in. We were able to move back into my house just four days before Christmas. It was hectic beyond belief. Apart from Margaret's machines, the large cutting table and rolls of material; we had two of everything as far as furniture went. We decided my three piece suite was better than theirs, as mine was only six months old, and so they left their suite behind in the house for the next tenants. We had two fridge freezers, two washing machines, two tumble dryers, three double beds and two single beds. We had no choice other than to give away what we couldn't use. There was no time to sell anything. Margaret tried to hang on to her dish washer, which had to go outside because there was no room for it, but eventually she had to give that away as well. Everything had happened so fast, otherwise it would have meant paying another six months' rent on the other house for the sake of two weeks.

There was a real feeling of home now, but despite the fact that I was much happier, I still had terrible nightmares from which I couldn't wake. I was forever shouting out in my sleep and never seemed to have nice dreams anymore. My hand was still shaking and my body was jerking more than ever now, and what doesn't show to others is the trembling inside of me, around my organs. It felt as if my whole insides were shaking . . . a feeling that is impossible for me to explain. Parts of me appear to have a life of their own and I can't control them. Because of the shaking in my hand, it takes a long time for me to fasten buttons and dressing seems to take for ages. Tying up shoe laces is impossible. Velcro shoes are a godsend, although I didn't like the idea of them at first, thinking they were like children's shoes. Something else was happening to me . . . every morning my pillow was wet from my drooling during the night. I constantly had to keep a handkerchief at hand because I was making so much saliva.

Are these Symptoms of Parkinson's disease, or the effects of the medication?

Chapter Four

Happy Days

(2004)

Looking back, I have to say that apart from my having Parkinson's disease, and the side effects of the medication, I believed things couldn't be any better than they were. This was the happiest I had felt since Joyce had died, and it was good to have people in the house again. I felt I could cope with my illness now I wasn't alone. The very first thing Margaret and Geoff did was to register with a new doctor, registering myself at the same time. The surgery was the same one Margaret had tried to get me and Joyce to join all those years ago. Here the doctors and staff were so different to the ones I'd been used to, and everyone was polite and friendly, plus it was only a short walk from the house. On my first visit the doctor shook my hand and introduced himself, and each and every time I went to the surgery, the doctors were all very pleasant. I was never made to feel rushed or flustered. The difference was amazing. Margaret was right; the majority of doctors are different to the ones I had been used to. Perhaps Joyce would still have died from Cancer, had we changed doctors, but at least she would have been treated with more respect. I can hear her now.

'Paddy, I'm going to have to go to the doctor's, this pain in my shoulder is killing me, I can't stand to move my neck. This isn't arthritis. I wish someone would listen to me. It's such a long walk up to the surgery and my whole body aches.'

'Shall I ring the doctor and ask him to come out'

'He won't come out. He wouldn't come out the last time. The receptionist said it wasn't an emergency. But I'm going to have to walk up there and ask for something stronger for this pain.'

'It would be better if the surgery was much further away, at least we could catch a bus.'

'I'd be willing to catch the bus, even if it was only just one stop away, but the buses don't go near the surgery, and we can't afford a taxi.'

Oh Joyce! I wish we could go back in time.

*

There were many changes taking place in the house. I had moved into the back bedroom, so Margaret could use the biggest bedroom for sewing. My room had been decorated using bright colours, with posh looking curtains that Margaret made, called 'Swags and Tails.' Everything looked and worked really well, except when I was getting dressed. I was having difficulty bending down to put my shoes on. Time and time again, I slipped off the edge of the bed, until one day Margaret came rushing upstairs when she heard a thud.

'Dad, why are you sat on the floor with your foot in the air holding a sock on your toes?

'I er . . . fell off the bed trying to put my socks on.'

Her eyes rolled towards the ceiling, as she laughed and helped me up. Within days I was bought a low chair for my bedroom. Now I could put my shoes and socks on with ease, which was much better than losing my balance and falling off the bed. The original separate toilet and bathroom had been made into one big bathroom, which Geoff had completed when he stayed in the house on his own. It was surprising how much bigger this made the bathroom. Now I could use a chair when I was getting shaved.

Each morning, either Margaret or Geoff would bring me a cup of tea, giving me time to come round, and allow my medication time to work before I got out of bed. I actually looked forward to getting up in the mornings, and I enjoyed my breakfast again as I had in the past. The house was full of homely smells once more from cooking and baking . . . in fact the whole atmosphere of the house had changed, turning it into a happy home again.

Geoff was usually out working during the day. He had a lot of travelling to do as most of his work was thirty or forty miles away in North Yorkshire, and this meant I spent a lot of time with Margaret. She used the front bedroom to work from, being the largest of the upstairs rooms, but being a north facing room the light wasn't very good after midday, and she always made sure she got a good early start in the morning. While she was working, I would vacuum the carpets, dust the furniture, and wash the breakfast dishes while listening to the radio; which seemed to play happier songs. I kept Margaret supplied with cups of tea or coffee, sitting at the side of her while she did her sewing, just as I had done when she ran her soft furnishing shop. We often talked about the plans Geoff had for the house and garden, and I was looking forward to the summer. Some days we walked up to the shops to get some cakes from the bakery, and ate them after lunch when she was having a break. There was nothing wrong with my appetite now, I enjoyed every meal and I drank sensibly.

One morning, while we were still living in Cottingley waiting to move into my house, Margaret had brought up the subject of alcohol. 'I don't think we should have any whisky in the house anymore Dad. It isn't good for you, and it's time to get it all out of your system. Stick to a couple of cans a lager a night instead . . . look here, I have some photos to show you.'

The photographs were taken during the summer months a couple of years ago. There were quite a few of me, taken down by the canal and some in the shop. Margaret then showed me the latest photos taken of me. I was shocked to see my face, red from whisky drinking, and swollen to the point where my eyes seemed to have disappeared. I looked like an alcoholic. I was more than happy to give up whisky after seeing those photographs.

Being able to have a conversation is another great pleasure after spending all those days on my own. It's hard to believe that I once liked to talk for hours at a time. *Nonstop Walt,* Joyce used to say. I would talk all the way through a film and she would yell "For God's sake Paddy, shurrup, I'm missing half of the film". I would go very quiet and she would smile at me and say "Put kettle on Paddy".

Margaret surprised me one day by asking if I believed in the afterlife. I paused awhile.

'Yes. I do. I didn't always believe in life after death. Not even after hearing all those Irish tales of spirits when I lived in Dominick Street. Jaysus, when I was a lad, the Irish loved a good get together. My grandmother, known as The Nan, and Molly, a relative that lived above us in the tenement house, used to talk about the 'cry of the Banshee', a female spirit in Irish mythology known as an omen of death. According to Irish folklore, she would come to the window of the person who was about to die, combing her long wild hair, howling and laughing, showing off her witch like ugly features through the glass. They say the cry of the Banshee is an unearthly sound, that sends dogs and cats running for cover, but as I grew older I would laugh at these tales. But the thing is, I know I have seen Joyce. I know it was her who woke me the night I fell asleep in the chair, and I also know Joyce believed in life after death. I remember her saying to me a few weeks before she died, "it's only like going through a door into another room." Her eyes had lit up as she said, "me mam and dad will be waiting for me, and our Tom." I didn't think for one minute it was true, but the thought of seeing her mam and dad, and her brother Tom again made it easier for Joyce to accept she was dying, so I didn't say anything.'

'I know Dad. She told me the same thing. I suppose she had plenty of time to think of dying during all those months when she couldn't sleep for the pain.' Margaret said softly. 'She also reached out and shouted, "Mam" as if she had seen her mother not long before she passed away if you remember. We were all there at the time. She could definitely see someone in front of her. I had a dream about a year before me mam died. In my dream, I was sat at my machine, sewing in the shop, when I suddenly looked up to see the outer door flung open followed by the inner door, as if a blast of wind had blown in. but it wasn't the wind . . . it was me mam walking towards the desk, smiling at me. She looked young, beautiful and really happy. She told me in my dream that she was dead. It was awful; my pillow was wet through with tears. I told her about the dream the day after, and she said "I hope that wasn't an omen". I didn't understand what she had meant at the time and we laughed it off.'

'Yes, she was really superstitious. She didn't like birds flying in the house, because apparently, it was a sign of death, so when a robin flew into the kitchen one day she was mortified; even more so when a week later a picture fell off the wall. Straight away, she said "I hope that's not for me." Don't be silly Joyce, I said, it's only a superstitious old wives tale. Pictures do fall of walls sometimes.'

'What do you mean? Is that a sign of death as well Dad?' Margaret asked.

'Supposedly . . . so is hearing a dog howl in the night. Joyce believed in that sort of thing. But, the point is, she knew she was going to die, long before she was diagnosed and sent home time and time again with a prescription for Irritable Bowel Syndrome. She showed me how to use the washing machine and peg clothes on the line. Little things like that, as if she was thinking about how I would cope without her.'

'They do say people know Dad, and if you remember, there was a certain sadness and gloom hanging in the air, as if something awful was about to happen. No one said anything, but I suppose it's like the shadow of death lurking in the background. Yet, we never knew how seriously ill she was at the time. Look at the missing pillow case. That was weird.'

When Joyce was first taken into hospital, Margaret thought she would surprise her by making new curtains, a valance and matching bedding for our bedroom. We spent a day cleaning the windows and putting the curtains and valance up, and madding my bed. When it came to putting the matching pillow slips on the bed, there was one missing. We couldn't find it anywhere. "Dad, I remember putting the two pillows slips in the bag." We searched the room and the bedding we had taken off to look for it. Margaret looked in the car, but it wasn't there. My side had a new pillow slip and Joyce's didn't. I had the most awful sense of dread inside me, and from the quietness I knew Margaret also had the same thought. The following day she was back again with another pillowcase she had made that morning. We took some photos of the room and showed them to Joyce. She held them against her chest and a tear fell down her cheek.

She knew she wasn't coming home.

'I had a strange dream once' I said to Margaret 'although I don't believe it was a dream really. I'd been having a lot of pain in my chest all week and put it down to indigestion. I woke up to reach over to the bedside cabinet for an antacid tablet, and I was conscious of the bedroom door opening slowly, letting the light from the landing shine through. I turned my head to look and saw a young girl about the age of nine or so, and at first my mind slipped back a few years and I thought it was you. She seemed to glide past me towards the foot of the bed. She was dressed in a white flowing dress that seemed to ripple as if a breeze was gently blowing. Her hair was long and black, which was why I thought it was you, and her piercing blue eyes were looking straight into mine. I suddenly realised, the light I had believed to come from the landing was actually coming from the girl herself. She was smiling and beckoning me to go to her. Of course I tried to shake yer mam, who was sleeping beside me, but found I couldn't move. I was completely paralysed. I tried shouting her name, but found I couldn't speak either; nothing would come out of my mouth. I panicked as the girl stood at the foot of the bed, holding out her hands to me. Jaysus . . . there was such a calm serene feeling in the room; it made me want to go to her. I don't know how I knew, but if I went with the girl I wouldn't come back. I was tempted, but I thought of yer mam sleeping beside me, and knew I couldn't leave her or my kids. I managed to close my eyes tight shut and when I opened them the girl was gone. Shaking and sweating, I managed to wake Joyce, who was more concerned about the way I looked than wanting to hear of the girl. The pain in my chest had returned, but it was much more painful than it was earlier.'

'Didn't me mam feel anything when she woke up?'

'No, at least I don't think so. She phoned for an ambulance, and I was rushed into hospital where I had a massive heart attack, and was critically ill for three days, as you know. Jaysus! I remember thinking, *was I supposed to die? Was it my time to go? Had the girl come to collect me? Or was it one of those so called near death experiences?* I've heard people say when you die; a loved one comes to take you to the 'other side'. For years after the dream, I wondered why a young girl would be the one to come for me. But eventually, I remembered when my baby sister, who incidentally had dark hair and blue eyes, died at the age of ten months, and my aunt Sissy saying to me. "Paddy, yis will have a guardian angel by your side fer the rest of yer life." So I suppose it must have been my sister. You see, although I was only young at the time, I carried her coffin through the streets of Dublin with my stepfather. Women didn't attend a child's funeral in those days. They stayed at home with relatives, and the child was taken to a special place where all the babies were buried together.'

We spoke of many things, and these conversations went on daily as we talked about the past, the present and the future.

*

Margaret stayed on the hypnotherapy course until after Christmas, and when she had qualified; she put an advertisement in the local paper. She named her new business 'Atlantis Hypnosis' and almost immediately, she was taking on clients and keeping busy. It was a good time to make changes, as January was a quiet time for both making and fitting curtains. Geoff hadn't much work on either, so it was also a good time to work on the conservatory. It didn't take very long to build, and once completed Margaret worked from there as a clinical hypnotherapist. She soon felt confident enough to rely solely on her hypnotherapy practice, and as her hands were beginning to trouble her due to all of the sewing over the years, she decided to stop sewing altogether and become a full time hypnotherapist.

It was probably about the same time Margaret gave up sewing when I started to have a problem showering. Up to then I had managed all right, although I had to be careful as the shower was over the bath. I was gradually finding it harder to hold on to something to keep my balance, and decided it might be better to bathe now rather than shower. Unfortunately, this was no easy task either. Climbing into the bath was fine, but it was a nightmare climbing back out again. I told Margaret of my situation, and she phoned Social Services to see if they could help. Within a few days a bath chair was installed over the bath, but although the idea was good, it wasn't really suitable for someone who has Parkinson's; my muscles were too stiff and of course my hand still shook. The occupational therapist came out to weigh the situation up once more, and made arrangements for a bar to be installed on the bath for me to grab a hold of. However, I was taking a bath one evening, when I couldn't get out. My legs were too rigid.

I lay there for a while. I couldn't shout for Margaret for obvious reasons, but as luck would have it, I heard the sound of Geoff's voice. This had to be the most embarrassing moment ever for me. Geoff couldn't lift me out of the bath, not without me getting my feet down securely, which I couldn't do. I was extremely stressed, which made the shaking in my arm increase. Geoff, on seeing my distress, had to admit defeat and phone my grandson, Michael, a strong, well build man, who lives nearby. Much to my relief . . . the water being cold by now, Michael was able to come right away. Together they lifted me out of the water and sat me on a chair. I was wrapped in a large towel, shivering and embarrassed by the fact that I had been stuck in the bath. I was really glad it was all over.

The next day Geoff rang Social Services to ask for information about having a wet room built in the old wash house, which was downstairs. We never thought for one minute there would be a problem; it was, after all, a genuine reason. Besides which, there was hot and cold water, and drainage already in situ. We were shocked to hear it would take months to make the application and wait for a decision, and even longer still before being able to put the shower in. How was I supposed to keep clean until then? Would I have to wait a year or more to take a shower?

In desperation, the very next day Geoff took a sledge hammer to the dividing wall between the wash house and the downstairs toilet.

Within a couple of weeks he had built a walk in shower cubicle, big enough for me to sit on a special chair, and room enough for him to help if need be. The bathroom looked lovely when the tiles on the walls and floor were fitted. The sea green colours of the curtains and towels matched, and candles were added. Joyce would have loved it. I was advised by Margaret and Geoff to only shower when Geoff was at hand, and as he works flexible hours, my showers were often at different times of the day. But at least I had a shower.

It was embarrassing at first, having my son-in-law in the room where I showered, but he soon put me at ease.

'We've both been in the forces Paddy. We've seen it all before and it's only the same as a male nurse helping you to shower.'

Oh Jaysus, I remember the forces. I was in the Irish Army. Curragh camp it was, in County Kildare and the place where I did my square bashing. Those barrack blocks held no privacy, as over twenty of us slept in the same room. Side by side we slept, with just a locker and a narrow wardrobe to divide your own space from that of the next man. I remember one of the lads keeping us awake night after night, grinding his teeth in his sleep; Jaysus that was the most awful sound. Just as we thought the grinding had stopped, it would jolt us out of our sleep again. It reached the point where we were waiting for it to happen and couldn't sleep at all. Each night someone would throw a boot at the poor lad, who obviously couldn't help himself.

'Jesus holy mother of God' he would shout, 'how am I supposed to know what I do in my sleep fer Christ's sake. If yis were to go to sleep in the first place, yis wouldn't be woken up by me.'

Now that took some working out, but I'm ashamed to say, I was one of the men that would throw something at him; though not a boot. Of course there were other heavy snorers who also had objects thrown at them, but the terrible grating sound of teeth was by far the worst.

When you went to the toilet block, to do your ablutions, only narrow flimsy screens separated you from all the other men who were trying to ignore everyone else. Geoff was right, it didn't take you long to adapt in those circumstances.

Later on in my training I was posted to the Dublin barracks, right in the heart of the City, where I was to set out and serve at table in the officer's mess. In comparison to the Curragh camp these buildings were built from grey stone. Huge imposing structures standing solidly along the banks of the River Liffy; where hundreds of men lived side by side in the bleak and depressing barrack blocks. Our barracks were a far cry from the splendour and comfort of the officer's mess, which was situated in the main area that flanked the parade square. It was on this parade ground where we would practice marching. Backwards and forwards, to and fro, up and down we would march. 'Bye the left, quick march.' Swinging our arms in unison, we would pace out the steps that were being measured by the Drill Sergeant, as he placed his yard stick on the ground as if it was a measuring stick. In and out, we would weave as we reached the boundaries of the parade square. With eyes faced forward and chin held firmly in, no one dared to glance to the side for fear of being put on a charge, until eventually we would practice with the band. I remember that parade. We marched around Phoenix Park which, at 1,750 acres, is one of the largest walled city parks in Europe. My mother was somewhere in the crowd, but I had to keep looking straight ahead. She was very proud of me in my uniform, but when I went home on leave I was given a telling off for not waving to her.

Geoff had been in the Royal Air Force and he talks to me while I shower. He talks about his life and the time he was in the forces. How he learned all the trades that would help him put the extensions onto the house. I'm grateful to him for helping me keep clean. It would be unthinkable to go a day or two without a shower. In fact, Margaret used to say to me years ago before we all lived together.

'Every time I phone you Dad, you're either in the shower, about to go in the shower or you have just got out of the shower.'

Now when I'm finished in the bathroom, I have a cup of tea while I sit on a chair wrapped in a warm towel to give me a breather, before I continue to get dressed.

Geoff had already drawn up plans to build a large therapy room for Margaret, instead of a sewing room as previously intended. It was to be the full length of the house, complete with a bathroom. Geoff showed me the plans when they were finally finished.

'It's a therapy room for Margaret, but there's plenty of extra insulation to keep it warm during the winter, and I'm putting French doors in. If it gets to a stage when you can't get upstairs, this can always be a bedroom for you. There's going to be plenty of room when I link the washhouse onto the extension, and then you will have your own en-suite shower room. The old coal house is large enough to make into a walk in wardrobe. So there will be plenty of space, and it will make a lovely downstairs bedroom. . . not that I'm thinking in terms of the near future, it could be years from now, but at least it will all be ready for you.'

Jaysus, I hope it never gets to that stage, I like my own bedroom. "Coal house?" I can't put my clothes in a coal house, and I couldn't sleep downstairs, especially in a room with French windows that used to be a garden. Does this mean my condition is going to get to the stage where I cannot walk and I will need wheelchair access?

I loved my bedroom upstairs with all the bright colours and didn't like to complain, but I was having trouble getting out of bed. Try as I might, to sleep near the edge, I rolled backwards into the centre. Eventually I told Geoff.

'It's the mattress you and Joyce slept on, you've both probably slept nearer the middle and it's sunk a bit. I'm working tomorrow so I'll ask Margaret to take you for a new mattress.'

I must have tried a dozen mattresses in various shops. The one I decided to buy was an anti-roll mattress, the one with the hippopotamus on the label. Right from the start I hated it. A week later I had to tell Margaret.

'What's wrong with it Dad? It's an anti-roll mattress; it's supposed to stop you rolling into the middle.'

'But it's hard and I like soft mattresses.'

'You must have known it was hard when you tried it out in the shop.'

'I was getting fed up by that time, and I thought it would do. Another thing; I keep falling off the edge when I sit on the bed. It's too stiff, it doesn't sink down.'

'The mattress was really expensive, and they won't take it back now you have slept on it for a week. You should have said you were fed up of trying beds out. We could have gone back the day after.'

'I know. I'm sorry.'

'It doesn't matter. I suppose we can use that one, and get rid of ours. Perhaps a single bed might be better for you now Dad, but we'll have to get a new one; we need the other single beds for when the kids come to stay. You'll have plenty of room to move about in the bedroom as well, with a single bed.'

And so we were shopping again, and this time we bought a single bed. A few days later I had to break the news to Margaret that the bed was too high.

'I can hardly climb onto it. The mattress is too thick. Come and see for yourself, I'll show you.'

She sighed and followed me upstairs and I struggled to climb onto the bed. She agreed with me, and said she would have a word with Geoff as to what we could do. Geoff was home early in the afternoon and he took a look at the bed. He worked some measurements out from the height of the bed and my legs. It took a while but he made some calculations and sawed the pine legs down to make them shorter. Now I could climb in and out easily.

A few months went by and I was having problems sitting from a lying position, so I was bought a big wedged pillow. This didn't solve the problem, so Geoff got in touch with the occupational therapist again. A woman came out to install a bed riser that fitted under the mattress, and raises the bed when you press a button. It wouldn't work because the mattress was too thick and being new, it wouldn't bend, so Geoff suggested she left the bed riser with us, and we bought a memory foam mattress that bent easily. At last progress was being made.

'Dad, you're like flipping Goldie Locks. You've had more beds in a month than we've had in ten years.'

'There's a thing; I haven't had any porridge for years.' I joked.

'I don't know how me mam put up with you.' Margaret laughed 'I'll get you some porridge tomorrow.'

It didn't end there. The mattress was very warm and because of my night sweats, I was bought a lighter weight duvet instead of the warmer duvet. But then my feet were too cold, so Margaret bought me a few lightweight blankets to cover the bottom half of the bed. The single mattress was used to replace one of the single beds in the back bedroom, which was the boy's room when they came to say, and the older mattress was taken to the tip.

At last I could sleep properly.

Once the plans had been passed, the building work for the extension began and I was envious of Geoff, watching him mix the concrete for the foundations and the mortar for the brickwork. I really wished I was able to help him. I knew how . . . being in the building trade for most of my working life, but at least I was able to watch. It seemed strange to see the whole house expand. Things were changing fast. Now, we have a bay window, a porch and a much bigger kitchen; I hardly recognise my home of fifty years. Later, I was encouraged by Geoff to help lay the Patio, and this gave me great satisfaction. We used small blocks that were light to lift, making patterns around the larger paving slabs that Geoff had laid.

The house was finished in no time. Margaret's therapy room was complete and she had a good little business. Unfortunately for me, she didn't have the same time to sit and talk as we had before, and I missed those days. But at least she was always at home. When she was busy with someone, I would take the phone calls from would be clients, and write their name and number down on a card at the side of the phone. Some days she might only have the one client, or even none at all, and we would meet Teresa and have a day in town shopping. She taught me how to e mail my brother, Michael, in Ireland. A computer must be the nearest miracle to electricity being discovered. Here I was, talking to my brother through a machine that sent the message within seconds . . . and I didn't even need a stamp!

The extension stretched the whole side of the house and clients could come and go through the French doors at the front. Geoff had put wood flooring down in the new room. He hadn't liked it much, as I hadn't, but Margaret said it was trendy and easier to clean, and so it was. There were diplomas and certificates across one wall from all of the courses she had been on. One course seemed to be a reason to start another course. 'Holistic therapies' she had told me. She used to spend a lot of time in her new room, either with a client or working on the computer, and one day I heard her talking to someone on the telephone. All of a sudden there was a loud crashing sound. I slowly got up from my chair and went to see what the noise was. Margaret was laid on the floor with her head under the desk, flat out with her eyes closed. I was getting used to all these weird therapies she was up to, including meditation and something called Reiki, which sounded like a gardening tool, and so I went back to my chair. A few minutes later, Margaret walked into the room, white as a sheet and holding the back of her head. I asked if she was all right. Half laughing and half crying, she replied.

'No. Not really. I've just fallen backwards off the chair, banging my head on the edge of the desk and then again on the floor. I feel sick and I have a massive headache. The chair just slid from under my feet. I was aware of you walking in the room and I tried to speak to you, but you walked out again. Didn't you wonder why I was lying on the floor?'

'No', I said, 'I thought you were asleep or something.'

'Dad, I could have been in a coma and you thought I'd taken a nap under the computer desk.'

'Well, you're always doing things like meditation and stuff so I didn't want to disturb you. Are you all right? Shall I make you some tea?'

'No, I think I should go and get it checked out at the hospital. I really did see stars. I've probably fractured my skull.'

She reached for her bag and keys and yelled 'shan't be long Dad . . . don't open the door to anyone while I'm out.'

She drove to the hospital to make sure she was all right, and was told she had concussion. She was given a slip of paper which told her to watch for sickness and severe headaches, and was told off for driving to the hospital herself.

Within weeks the wooden floor was replaced with a carpet. It was just as well. Apart from Margaret's accident, Bonny's legs would slide in all directions when she ran to greet people who were coming through the door. She looked like Scooby Doo, and it was only a matter of time before I would have slid myself. Sometimes I was finding it hard to lift my feet as I walked and believe me, I was glad to see the back of the wooden floor. It was cold looking and reminded me of the days when we couldn't afford carpets for the bedrooms.

Geoff, eager to start work on the garden now spring was here, soon built a pond which was quite big with a little waterfall where birds came to bathe every morning. The lovely sound of birds singing was delightful. Bushes, trees and flowers were planted, and I was shocked when they told me some of the plants were put there because they attracted bees. Joyce was terrified of bees. She would never have gone outside. I soon learned that if the bees were left alone, they didn't bother anyone. From trying to swat bees and kill them for all those years, I was now encouraged to protect them!

*

I was walking into the kitchen from the lounge, when suddenly Margaret's voice startled me. 'Dad, stand up straight and lift your head up. Come on, I know stiffness is a symptom of Parkinson's disease, but it doesn't mean to say we have to conform and give in to it. Have a good stretch and push those shoulders back and stop shuffling your feet.'

I wasn't aware of walking with my head down, but I straightened myself up as best I could. I knew my posture wasn't as good as it used to be, I had seen my reflection in shop windows when I was in town. I was to hear those words time and time again.

'Come on Dad, shoulders back, lift your head up. March on the spot, lift those legs. You're shuffling again.'

I would stand there marching up and down to Margaret's orders.

'Up two three four, up two three four, you're in the Army now lad, get marching, up two three four, lift those knee's lad, lift those knee's. Swing those arms, one two three, one two three.'

She would do the march with me and then we would flop onto the settee laughing, exhausted.

Margaret's 'bullying' continued for years to come, and she managed to make sure I exercised every day during those early years of Parkinson's disease. This probably helped tremendously, as I didn't lean to one side as much as I used to, and I managed to lift my feet when walking.

To help me even further, a letter arrived asking me if I wanted to go to physiotherapy classes. It was a twelve week course and I really enjoyed it. To help our reflexes we played silly games, such as throwing a ball to each other without warning, and games like 'Guess Who' to exercise the brain or as Margaret called it 'The cognitive bit.' We had to mimic someone famous during one of the sessions, and I had the nurses laughing, because I mimicked Charlie Chaplin and took him off very well. I showed my walk to

Margaret when I came home, and she was in stitches laughing at me swinging my walking stick, with my legs closed tight together.

Over the weeks, we learned easier ways of fastening buttons and the fiddly things of getting dressed. This was really helpful because my hands were getting stiffer as each day passed. It could take me a while to get dressed and undressed, but I needed to keep my independence as long as possible, and I kept it to myself for as long as I could. We were taught how to use a walking stick properly, to make it work for you, and how to walk up and down steps with it. We also baked at the centre, and I would make cakes or pies to bring home for Bonny and me. She always recognised the sound of the transport bus driving up to the house even before it stopped. Bonny would race down the path, her tail wagging in the air as she ran to greet me. Her head would go straight to the bag which was in my hand to see what I had made that day. The staff gave us exercises to do at home and I tried to do them every day, I had no other choice. Margaret wasn't going to let me forget to do them.

'Have you done your exercises today Dad? Keep it up, don't you be getting old and stiff now.'

My speech seemed to have become very quiet, and I forever had to repeat myself to be heard. After an appointment at the Parkinson's clinic, at Margaret's request, I was sent to see a speech therapist at the hospital. It took ages to find the department. The therapy clinic is a building on the outside of the hospital, and on the way there I bumped into a nurse from the physiotherapy class. She flung her arms around me, much to the amused look on Margaret's face.

'Patrick. How lovely to see you. How are you? I haven't seen you for a while. I was on holiday when you last came to physiotherapy. Are you all right?'

She told Margaret how I made the nursing staff laugh every time I was there, "what, with that cheeky Irish humour of his".

We stood talking to her for a while and said our goodbyes. She gave me a big hug. Margaret was laughing at me on the way to the Speech therapist's office.

'You're a right little charmer, you are. All the nurses at the hospital remember you. A nurse even stopped to speak to you in the hospital restaurant. "Once seen, not forgot" as me mam used to say . . . and who was that you were talking to in Wallis's the other day, the young girl who was serving?'

'She used to work at the post office and help me choose birthday cards.'

I smiled. It was true, the staff always remembered my name, and the nurses at the day care unit were very pleasant to me. Sadly, you were only allowed the one twelve week course, as there was a waiting list for new patients. Those were happy times. Unfortunately, a few years later, I heard a nurse saying to Geoff that they don't have classes at all now because of the cuts to services. That was such a shame; it was very helpful and educational for me at that time in my life, and being with others who have the same problems was also good for me.

This was to be the one and only time that I saw a speech therapist. It seems there is no follow up or checking system to see if a patient needs help in the future, even though difficulties with speech is quite common for people with Parkinson's. When I first went to see the therapist, my speech wasn't too bad and I could speak up if I really tried, but as time went by, it was an effort to keep up with conversations.

These were happy days, but unfortunately, it wasn't to be long before Parkinson's disease reared its ugly head. The best years of my life, since losing Joyce, were soon to be a thing of the past.

Chapter Five

Changing Times

(2006)

The first few years after being diagnosed with Parkinson's disease had gone by without a great deal of change, and I remember thinking if this was all there was to it, I could cope. But that was not to be. My hand was shaking a lot more now, and the jerking inside of my body was driving me mad. I was really struggling with the simplest of tasks, such as getting dressed in a morning, shaving and even cutting into my food. My neck was very stiff and much worse; I seemed to rest my head to one side when sitting, or nodding off to sleep.

One day I was woken by such a commotion. 'Oh my god . . . Geoff, come quick' Margaret screamed 'me dads passed out.'

I opened my eyes and wondered why I was nearly on the floor upside down. I must have fallen asleep, and slowly leaned over to a point where the top half of my body had slid over the chair arm. Geoff sat me up and Margaret walked over to ask if I was all right.

'You scared the life out of me, I thought you were dead.'

'I didn't know I had fallen . . . and I didn't know I was asleep, it's those tablets.'

'Well, next time try to sit up straight before you nod off. Don't be scaring me like that.'

'That's the problem; I don't know I'm falling asleep. It's the tablets.'

'I know you keep saying it's the tablets, but you have to take them. I think we're going to have to get you a chair with wings at the side.'

'I might fly away then instead of falling.'

'Yeah, you probably would.' she laughed 'I think perhaps we ought to be looking at buying a chair which will stop you leaning to the left. One that's a little higher, to make it easier for you to . . .'

'An old folks chair you mean? I'm not ready for one of those yet.'

'No, not an old folks chair particularly, but a nice comfortable chair with sides to stop you leaning. We can look at some tomorrow, it won't hurt to look.'

The next day Margaret took me to a disability shop that sold rise and fall chairs. We looked at all the range they had on show, and I was aghast at the prices, which ranged from £1,200 upwards. I could hardly believe it, my three piece suite didn't cost that much. I immediately pulled Margaret to one side.

'Jaysus, I can't believe how expensive they are. The cheapest one is £1,200. I don't think I need one really. I can manage with the one I have.'

Margaret agrees the chairs are expensive, and tells the salesman we will think about it before making a decision. We drove back home and she looked on the computer to find somewhere else that sold similar chairs. Eventually, she found a manufacturer in town which also sold direct to the public, and with my feet scrapping on the floor, I reluctantly went with her. Unbelievably, the prices were the same as the other shop, even though they made them. Margaret saw the look on my face.

'You do need a better chair Dad. Just think, you can recline it, and have a nap in the afternoon without getting a stiff neck. The chair rises to help you get out, and you can also raise your feet without lying down. You really do need a good chair Dad. You were upside down when you fell to one side. You could have hurt yourself.'

Paying out all that money for one will hurt me more.

Margaret knew exactly what I was thinking. 'You can afford it Dad, what's the point of saving money in the bank now. It's time you spoiled yourself. You can afford to buy one or two luxuries from your pension now we live with you. You don't have to worry about paying bills anymore. Treat yourself.'

'Yeah but I was saving the money for you all to share out when I'm gone.'

'Well, you're not going anywhere for a few years. You've plenty of time left, and you need to spend it on yourself. I'm sure the others would agree with me. After all, you've struggled all your life, you deserve to treat yourself. In any case, the amount of money you do have saved won't go very far when shared out between the five of us. Get the chair.'

I tried sitting in one particular chair which was very comfortable, but priced at £1,400. There was no way I was going to buy a chair at that price. I was just about to say so, when a lady approached us, dressed in a black suit, looking as if she was on her way to a funeral.

'I noticed you looked quite pleased with the chair you were looking at just now.' She said to Margaret.

'Yes, my father looked comfortable in it. Sometimes he has difficulty standing up from a sitting position. But they are all very expensive, so we need to discuss things and perhaps come back later.'

I noticed she didn't embarrass me by saying I was leaning to the left, which was a relief.

'Before you go, let me show you a chair we have in the back room. It's the same as this one, but much cheaper.'

We followed the lady to what seemed like a store room, and she walked towards a chair which was exactly the same as the one out in the showroom.

'An elderly lady bought this chair six weeks ago, but as her legs were a little short, she couldn't cope with it. Her son brought it back, but unfortunately, we couldn't refund him the full amount of money as it's really second hand now.' She showed us the ticket that was still beneath the chair to prove how 'new' it was. 'We gave him a refund of £800, and as we don't really sell second hand furniture, I can let you have it for the same amount if you want it.'

Of course, Margaret jumped at the chance and agreed to take the chair. On the way home she asked me if I was looking forward to sitting in it.

'I bet you can't wait for the chair to come tomorrow, talk about home comforts. It was a good deal that Dad, wasn't it?'

'No. I think the old woman died in it.'

'What makes you say that?' Margaret asked, 'Her son lost £600 in six weeks and the shop could have refused to take it back.'

'If that's true, why didn't her son sell it for a higher sum to someone else? . . . I know why.'

'Go on then, why?'

'He wanted to get rid of it quick because she died in it. He couldn't stand it being in the house long enough to sell it, so he took it back to the shop.'

'Don't be silly Dad; it was because she was too small for it. Her feet wouldn't reach the floor.'

'She must have known that before she bought it.'

'Her son might have just gone out and bought it for her.'

'If that's the case, why didn't he take it straight back the same day?'

'Oh, you are so strange sometimes; I very much doubt the old lady died in the chair.'

'Anyway, it's electric, I might get a shock. What if I spill tea over it?'

'They wouldn't sell them if there was a chance someone could be electrocuted, now would they?'

The chair arrived the day after, and I sat anywhere but on the chair. After much persuasion, three days later, I finally gave it a try and found it really comfortable, although it didn't stop me thinking of the old lady. Dead! In the very chair I was sitting in. Two or three weeks went by and I finally had to admit the chair did make life easier. It was extremely simple to get in and out of, and when I fell asleep, my head had somewhere to rest. I was fascinated by the remote control and the amount of movement I could get out of it. I raised my legs, lay back and rose up, but, one day I pressed the button a little too long and the chair rose so high, I slid to the floor onto my bottom. Margaret came rushing in to my shouts.

'Dad, are you all right. What are you doing on the floor?'

'The old woman pushed me off.'

'No she didn't. You've been playing with the control again and pushed yourself too far. There are no ghosts in that chair.'

'There is, and it's the old woman.'

'Well, there's never a dull moment with you. Fancy a cuppa?'

'Yeah' I replied sulkily.

'Does your friend, the old woman want one?'

'Ha-ha very funny. I'll ask her.'

*

I was preparing to leave for the hospital, when I looked into a mirror to check my tie, and wished I hadn't.

'My body looks twisted. Is it this coat? And my left shoulder is lower than my right. Does my face look different to you? It looks longer.'

'You look all right to me Dad, and still look as handsome as ever. Your coat just needs straightening up a bit. The mirror in this room isn't very flattering when the sun is shining.'

I knew she was just trying to make me feel better, but I know what I saw in the mirror . . . a twisted looking man with one shoulder higher than the other.

Six months had gone by since I had last been to the Parkinson's clinic, and we were on our way to another appointment to see the consultant at the hospital. It was Monday morning and very busy in the car park. After driving around the car park for about twenty minutes, trying to find a space, Margaret became frustrated.

'There's no room to park, so I'm going to park in an ambulance spot at the back of the hospital. It's nearer to the clinic, and it's only an ambulance car park for picking up and dropping off patients.'

This car park was also very busy, but eventually she managed to find a little spot to pull into.

'I'll drop you off here and take you into the clinic, otherwise we'll be late. I'll book you in and find a place to park in the main car park. Then I'll fetch the car when we come out.'

Margaret opened the door for me and helped me out of the car, and I stood waiting for her to lock the car doors. For some time I'd been having a problem with my left leg. It would spontaneously move across my right leg. This had happened a few times at home and I'd spun round and almost fallen down. As I stood there waiting, the very same thing happened. I spun almost all the way round and completely lost my balance, falling to the ground, right there in the road. Margaret was shocked and rushed to my side. She anxiously looked around for help, but there wasn't a person in sight.

'Oh my God, Dad what am I going to do? I can't leave you here while I go inside for help, someone might run over you when they turn the corner. They won't see you in time. I don't know what to do.'

She tried lifting me to a standing position, but I couldn't get my feet flat long enough to stand and help her, and I felt useless and angry with myself. This part of the hospital was situated at the back, and much quieter than the entrance at the front, which is outside the main casualty department.

Someone eventually came running over from a building across the road. She must have seen it happen through her office window. Asking if I was all right, the lady then went to get some help. Two nurses arrived and I was gently helped into a wheelchair and taken into the clinic. It seemed a while before Margaret came rushing in after parking the car and I could tell she was upset. She sat down beside me and her hands were still shaking. After an hour and a half of sitting in the waiting room I was finally taken to be weighed. On returning from the weighing room I could see Margaret sitting there, pale and still upset. I knew she would be blaming herself and she did.

'It's my fault Dad. I shouldn't have been rushing you. All that panic trying not to be five minutes late . . . and for what . . . to wait two hours to see the consultant.'

Here I was, everyone fussing me and asking if I was all right. Did I need a drink or anything? Nobody considered how Margaret must be feeling. In fact, a nurse told her it wasn't a good idea to make hospital appointments early in the day, because my medication wouldn't have had time to work.

'People who have Parkinson's disease need time to come round on a morning. Their tablets need to start working. You have to take this into consideration when you arrange to take your father anywhere.'

Margaret was clearly upset by this remark, and I'm surprised she didn't say anything. She was already blaming herself in the first place, without extra pressure being put on her. How was she supposed to know the medication doesn't work straight away, for God's sake? And why then, did the hospital book an early appointment, knowing I was there with Parkinson's disease? I suppose it's probably because the department was for stroke patients and not a Parkinson's clinic. The hospital didn't appear to have a Parkinson's clinic. There were plenty of brochures, leaflets and papers around the clinic for strokes, but there were no brochures or leaflets to do with Parkinson's disease. Margaret even asked at the desk for any available information, and she was told they hadn't got anything on Parkinson's. I saw people in the clinic walking with a stoop or in wheelchairs. One man was so badly bent that he couldn't lift his head, but I didn't see anyone who had trembling in their hands.

Did any of them have Parkinson's disease, or had they suffered a Stroke? If it is Parkinson's, will I become like that in time?

I was to find out many years later, that no two people with this disease are the same, and it doesn't just affect the elderly, although everyone at the clinic were roughly my age. Michael J. Fox, the actor who starred in "Back to the Future" was diagnosed with Parkinson's disease at the age of thirty, and like me, it started with a twitch in his finger and also like me, he turned to drink in the beginning. I hear he wrote a book called "Lucky Man". I have never had the chance to read it, but I heard it was very good, though I can't think why he thinks he's lucky. I certainly don't feel that way.

The consultant asked how I was keeping. He checked my hands and looked at my face, had me walk across the small room, and then gave me some more medication to help stop the jerking and the shaking in my left hand. I hadn't changed much really from the previous visit, although the shaking and jerking had got slightly worse. We had to make a follow up appointment and walk to the pharmacy department, waiting another twenty minutes before going back to the car park. Margaret insisted I'd walked far enough for one day and told me to rest while she ran down for the car. We were both glad it was all over with. On the way home we called into the doctor's surgery, but there was nothing about Parkinson's there either.

What the hell is Parkinson's disease and what happens? Will it get worse than it is now? What am I to expect? Am I to live just a short time?

Worse still, now I had more medication to take and get used to. I just hoped it would put an end to my shaking hand. Well . . . it wasn't just my hand; it was my whole arm now, which was much harder to hide. I try to hold it still as I had done before, but the shaking is too strong and makes my 'good' hand shake from the vibration. The only information I had to read was on a leaflet that came with the tablets, but reading all of the possible side effects made me want to put a gun to my head.

May cause dizziness or make you drowsy, can induce sickness or diarrhoea, constipation, hallucinations, and may also cause anxiety, depression, emotional distress and obsessive compulsive disorders. What the hell is obsessive compulsive disorder?

Eventually, a booklet and information came through the post about Parkinson's, but this confused and frightened me even more.

The new medication did slow down my shaking and stiffness, but the downside was that I was always sleeping. I could fall asleep at anytime during the day and I had terrible dreams. I also felt quite sick and my stomach was upset. My mind wasn't the same; I was becoming very suspicious of everyone. I was convinced there was a conspiracy against me and I believed people were whispering behind my back. Once I accused Margaret and Geoff of making fun of me. They were extremely patient and also very concerned. I was incredibly confused with my feelings. I suffered all kinds of emotions, especially guilt, after accusing the two people who cared for me twenty four hours a day, of something they had not done. They would never have made fun of me. I was frightened and felt very much alone with my negative thoughts. *Why was I feeling like this?* They had given everything up to take care of me, and included me in everything.

Geoff was starting to get more concerned about me when Margaret told him how I had been one day. He took out my new medication and looked at the leaflet, and read it to me.

'Taking this medication may cause delusions.'

'What are delusions?' I asked Geoff. 'I have never heard of them.'

Geoff explained that delusions were the irrational feelings I was experiencing due to the medication I was taking. He told me the medication was stopping me from making logical decisions. How I was thinking things were real, when normally I would never have thought they were; but the suspicions were still there, I didn't understand it all. I was suspicious of everyone I came into contact with, not just Margaret and Geoff, but the rest of the family too. I was hearing voices all the time, and believed someone was following me around. I was sure of it. I tried to persevere with the tablets, hoping it would sort itself out in time.

Something was taking over my mind. The pills were messing up my brain.

A week after seeing the consultant I received a letter from the hospital saying I was discharged. Margaret was furious because the consultant had said he would see us in six months time, and she had made the appointment at the desk . . . of course for a later time in the morning. She phoned the hospital immediately. Obviously I couldn't hear the other end of the conversation, but I heard Margaret.

'How can they discharge him' she said after telling the receptionist about the letter. There was a pause while the receptionist spoke. 'I don't believe it' Margaret said, in a way that put me in mind of Victor Meldrew. 'You're saying he's been discharged because there's been little change in him over the last year. He has Parkinson's disease and from what little information we know about it, it is not going to go away. What if something happens and we need to see a specialist? There's a six months waiting list. What if my dad's condition changes; there would be a six months delay. No one has explained anything to us about the disease. I would like you to make another appointment for six months time as usual. He is not going to be written off. We don't know who the hell to turn to when something new happens as it is. We have not been given any information to explain what's likely to happen next.'

An appointment was made for six months time and I was not discharged again.

71

*

I had been feeling weak and lethargic since being on my new tablets, and Margaret thought it would be a good idea to use a wheelchair until I got used to the medication. She said it was only for walks that were sometimes a little too far. We decided to try it out when we went into town, and parked in one of the car parks that are very near to the centre, but also up a steep hill.

'At least you won't have to walk back up Dad; I can push you up to the car park.'

I reluctantly settled in the chair, feeling small and inferior.

'I don't like this idea. I feel like a dwarf in here, and I'll be able to feel you looking at the back of my head.'

'Dad, it's only a trial, and I promise I won't look at your head. When we go off somewhere for the day, it might come in very handy. I'm not for one minute suggesting you use it all the time, but it's useful to keep in the car.'

I sat back as she started to push. We turned the corner from the car park and began to go down the slope.

'Oh my God Dad' Margaret shouted with a fear in her voice. 'I can't hold on, the chair is pulling me down the hill . . . . It's really hard to hang on to . . . and I can feel my feet slipping.'

I looked at the steep slope in front of me and visualised myself careering downhill, smashing through all the happy shoppers until I am killed; Margaret, lying on her back staring after me, her arms outstretched.

'Sorry Dad, I can't hold on and I can't it stop either, the pavement is wet . . . I'm going to have to crash into the edge . . . brace yourself.'

We crashed into the edge, and my knees were sore from the impact.

'It's no good. You're going to have to get out and walk.'

I jumped straight out the chair. I didn't need asking twice.

'Jaysus, I'm glad to have me feet on the floor again.'

'I've never pushed a wheelchair before. I thought it would be like pushing a baby in a pushchair.'

'Yeah . . . and how much does a baby weigh compared to an adult.'

'Don't rub it in. I just didn't think. The pavement is wet from the rain.'

'How could you possibly push me back up if you can't push me downhill?'

'It's easier to push uphill, you have strength behind you.'

There was a pub across the road from where we were, and I can imagine the drinkers had their best laugh of the day, and were eager to tell the missus when they went home.

The wheelchair was taken back to the car, and even without me sitting in it, Margaret struggled.

'They ought to give training to the people who have the job of pushing a wheelchair. The brakes are in the wrong place for a start, I couldn't take my hand off the handles to reach it. I could feel it pulling away from me. You are really lucky Dad. If I'd have let go you would have been killed, it's quite a deep slope. They ought to have a warning sign on them saying.

"DO NOT PUSH THIS WHEELCHAIR DOWNHILL WHEN
SOMEONE IS SITTING IN IT".'

'You should have told me to put the brakes on.'

'Oh yeah, we probably would have done a wheelie or something . . . I know you Dad.'

'Where are the brakes anyway?'

'They're near the wheels. They should be on the handle bars.'

'I'm not going in it again.'

'And I'm not pushing it again.'

'I told you I didn't need a wheelchair.'

'But you might one day, and your legs were feeling weak, you said so earlier, and I thought we could just give it a try.'

'I won't be trying it again.'

'No, and neither will I.'

*

When Margaret and Geoff came to live with me, Geoff had an estate car for his job and Margaret had a saloon car. As the years had progressed since being diagnosed, the stiffness in my neck was causing problems for me getting in and out of a car. I couldn't seem to bend far enough down and was always banging my head. As time went by and the problem got worse, Margaret decided to change her car for a four wheel drive, believing that would help. It wasn't too bad at first. She had bought a little step, to help me to climb in, which made things so much easier than bending down. Unfortunately I was still having trouble getting out of the car. In the beginning I was able to 'slide' out, but once, after nearly falling, I lost my confidence and began to struggle. For three weeks the three of us looked for a decent car; one that I was able to get in and out of. I was becoming agitated about climbing into cars just to find one that was suitable, but eventually we found the perfect car, a Vauxhall Zafira. There was plenty of headroom and it was not too high up from the ground. The downside was the price, Margaret and Geoff simply couldn't afford it.

A few weeks later Margaret was talking to my daughter, Teresa, about the situation. Teresa asked why we hadn't got a disability car as I was already claiming mobility allowance. Margaret told her that she needed a car for herself.

'There doesn't seem much point if I can only use it when Dad's in the car. I need it for myself as well.'

'Dad doesn't have to be in the car,' Teresa said, 'you can still use it on your own so long as you don't use the badges for parking when he's not with you.'

So that was it. We went to a mobility garage and chose the Vauxhall Zafira. Margaret was thrilled. Neither of them knew we were entitled to a disability vehicle that could be used as a family car; they just assumed that the disabled person had to be in the car when it was being driven. They were even more shocked to find out that the car came complete with full tax, insurance and repairs.

*

Taking Bonny for a walk in the field was becoming harder. I felt alright once I was outside. It was the motivation to get up from the chair in the first place that I found hard. I seem to have gone from feeling restless, and wanting to be on the go, to having no enthusiasm for anything; everything seemed too much effort. It must have been hard for Margaret and Geoff, because I was grumpy from feeling frustrated. There was another man inside my body taking my personality away from me, and I was also becoming very clumsy. It was all too easy for a glass to fall out of my hand, spilling the contents onto the floor. On one occasion, I was drinking a cup of tea while sitting in the chair, when my arm suddenly jerked spontaneously, splashing the tea all over my face and clothes. The force of the jerk was so strong that the tea flew across the room, hitting Bonny in the face. On hearing me shout, Margaret came rushing through the door and for some reason unknown to me, I blamed the dog.

'It was Bonny, she came running over and jumped up to lick my face and the tea spilled all over.' I explained, but Margaret burst into laughter.

'Dad, the poor dog is in shock as to why a cup of tea was thrown at her. She's never moved from that spot. Anyone would think we were going to yell at you for spilling a drink. Things like that don't matter. It can't be helped, and I expect there will be many more spills to come. I'll make you a fresh pot.'

We were all beginning to learn how to cope with new situations. I was adjusting to the changes Parkinson's disease was imposing on me, and Margaret and Geoff were trying to work out the best way to make life easier for me. It really had been a time for changes.

Chapter Six

Lost in France

(2006)

My Parkinson's symptoms seemed to have been pretty stable for a few months, and when summer arrived Margaret started talking about a holiday.

'We haven't had a decent holiday for a few years, and I think we should have one this year.' Margaret said, looking through a magazine. 'It'll be good for my dad as well. Perhaps we could take Nicolas and Antony with us. They're teenagers now, and will be able to help us with Dad to give us a break. What do you think?'

'Where were you thinking of going?' Geoff asked.

'I thought we could go to France. Dad won't be able to go on a plane now and I don't fancy going to the coast, we can go there anytime. It'll be nice to go to France; we loved it the last time we went.'

Brochures were sent for and before long, the holiday to France was booked. Margaret and Geoff preferred self-catering holidays, as they allowed time for sightseeing without having to rush back for mealtimes. They opted for a chalet overlooking a large lake in Northern France, telling me we would travel in the car and cross over on the ferry. We had the Vauxhall Zafira by then, and the car had seven seats, so there was enough space for all of us and for the wheelchair . . . if I needed it . . . which I hoped I didn't . . . and if I did . . . I hoped Geoff would push it.

Nicolas asked if he could bring his friend Ryan with him, and soon we were all set to go. A part of me was looking forward to the holiday, but the thought of all that travelling did worry me. My neck was so stiff and was causing pain down my spine. The stoop I now had, as slight as it was, seemed difficult to live with. I felt as though my head was too heavy for my shoulders and when walking, the pace at which my body allowed me to move forward, made me feel as though I was trying to walk through water. Whenever I sat for long periods I would lean to one side, and so it was arranged for me to travel on the right hand side of the car, just in case I leaned on the door and it opened. A couple of pillows were propped in place to prevent me leaning to the left, and we were off.

It rained heavily all the way down to the Port of Dover, and we were all relieved to stretch our legs on the boat. The crossing only took just over an hour, and I was dreading going back to the car to start the journey again. I felt incredibly stiff and my stomach hurt. Once again, I had that feeling of wanting to use the bathroom to pass water. My bladder always seemed to be full, even after I'd been to the toilet to empty it, and I'm not sure if it was the same problem as before. Or was it, as Geoff had said, a symptom of Parkinson's, which can have an effect on the bladder. On top of all that, I was also forgetting what I wanted to say and this was making me feel anxious.

We travelled through the night to get to the resort and arrived the following morning, after stopping for refreshments and to stretch our legs. The chalet was much smaller than it had looked in the brochure, and the rain hadn't stopped since we set off from home. Fortunately, the boys had a great time at the resort, canoeing in the rain for one thing, and coming back to the chalet looking as if they had literally fallen in the lake, their clothes being so wet. Unfortunately, for me, we had only been there a few hours and I was ready for home. The chairs and the settee were basic and uncomfortable without arm rests, and this caused problems with me falling over to one side. The chalet had a good area of land and plenty of garden furniture, and so the problem was soon solved as Geoff brought a decent sized garden chair, which had arm rests and an extra cushion, into the lounge for me to sit on. As the week continued, we decided where to go each morning, all depending on the weather, although, even when it rained it was still warm, and we had plenty of day trips. I have to say, by that time, I was beginning to enjoy myself. Despite my difficulty walking, and my memory not being as good as it used to be, I was still in control of my other faculties.

A dream of mine had always been to go to see the war graves in Normandy, and on our way there we passed several war cemeteries, before eventually coming to a large cemetery flying a German flag. The boys were fascinated by the German graves, and were amazed how young some of the soldiers had been. It was good to see how sad they looked when realising some of the soldiers were just a little older than themselves. They recognized the young men were someone's son, grandson or brother, just as our soldiers had been. The thing that really surprised me was that the headstones were black. All the other headstones we had seen, including, French, Italian, British and American were white. These black headstones seemed very dramatic and the silence was uncanny, not even the sound of a bird. Nicholas was really affected by the sight of so many grave stones commemorating the deaths of these young men. As I'd stood next to him, holding onto my walking stick, he'd looked at me and said quietly.

'I will never watch a war film in the same way again after coming here, Granddad Paddy. You don't realise they were just the same as our lads, and didn't deserve to die.'

We started our expedition once more and Geoff began to tell us a little about the area.

'This particular part of France is steeped in the history of both the First and the Second World Wars, and also from times much earlier in French history. The road we're on now, was known as the Chemin des Dames or the 'Ladies Path' because it had been constantly used by the daughters of the eighteenth century French King, Louis XV, as they travelled between a large chateau and their home in Paris.'

For miles we travelled on lonely lanes without passing another car, or seeing any form of civilisation. I was beginning to feel a little nervous about this; until we finally came across a war museum called 'Caverne du Dragon', which translates as the 'The Dragon's Cave', right in the middle of nowhere. This was to be the highlight of my first holiday abroad. Our tour guide spoke very good English and he welcomed us all. There were just the five of us and a young couple from Ireland, and before we went down to the cave, the guide made a point of thanking the British, and also the Irish soldiers, who had fought in both wars. He escorted us to a large lift where we descended into a complex system of manmade caves. The caves had been quarried by Catholic monks to get the stone to build the many churches and cathedrals all over Northern France, and they were unbelievably large. The guide explained that the French army had originally used the caves as a command post, but the German troops had quickly forced them out. Once installed, the Germans built a complex array of sleeping quarters, a chapel and a sick bay, and the museum had life size manikins posing as doctors and nurses, operating on the bloodied wounded soldiers, some with missing limbs.

The guide asked if it was alright to switch the lights out, to give us a feel of what it was like for the soldiers. The lights were suddenly switched off and the sound of guns firing, grenades going off, and men screaming, gave a realistic and frightening feel to the tunnels. Passageways had been dug that led to the outside of the hillside, where machine gun posts had been placed. When the machine guns were fired, flames would spit out from the hillside, and at night the flames would light up the whole area. It was these flames that gave way to the name 'Drachenhole' or the 'Dragons Lair' because the German soldiers thought it looked like Dragon's breath.

As we continued around the caves we were told of the effects the wars had had on the local area and how, even today, they were still finding unexploded bombs and ammunition. The guide explained, that when trying to make safe the surrounding hillsides, the live ammunition which was found had filled a local swimming pool until it was exploded safely. He went on to say how farmers were still digging up unexploded shells. I was shocked because when we had stretched our legs for a while earlier in the day, we had stopped at a village called Craonne; well, it used to be a village, now it's just a series of bomb craters, and the remains of the buildings that people had lived in. As soon as we'd parked up, the three boys were running around, jumping in the bomb craters and climbing the remnants of the stone walls. As an act of remembrance, the whole area had been turned into an arboretum by planting many different species of trees and bushes. There was a sense of beauty and serenity, as we'd walked the twenty minute long route that takes you through the demolished buildings, and alongside the original cemetery; where some of the existing graves of the villagers, and photographs in special display cases can still be seen.

I really enjoyed my visit to the Dragon's Lair, and not surprisingly, so did the boys. Everything had been done to make disabled access possible, and even when the walkways took a steep turn or moved from one level to another, there was always a ramp or small lift which could be used for a wheelchair. A great deal of care had been taken during the design of the route around the cave, and it crossed my mind that perhaps it was because so many war veterans came to visit, that all this care had been taken. Who would have thought an underground world, hidden from view, could bring back to life the sights and sounds of two world wars, and also have excellent wheelchair access?

When the tour was over, our guide made his farewells and we walked out toward to the blue sky which could be seen at the top of a long ramp. On the way there was small area which housed a television screen and we all paused to take a look. The film showed real live footage of a French soldier being tied to a wooden stake and shot for desertion. Suddenly we were brought back to the realities of war, and the excitement of the boys running around those bomb craters in the deserted village, was put into perspective.

There were plenty of castles which we would have liked to have visited, but I was unable to walk up the stairs and usually there was no wheelchair access, and apart from being very disappointed, I felt as if I was holding everyone else back. Though most of the time I was able to walk on the flat with the aid of my walking stick, we still needed to take the wheelchair if there was much walking to do, and in many ways, I was grateful for the wheelchair. The sores on my chest and stomach, caused by the seatbelts, hurt from travelling, and my bladder felt constantly full, but everyone was having a good time and I had no intention of spoiling the holiday by telling them of my discomfort.

*

The morning we went to Disneyland, the sun was shining and there wasn't a drop of rain all day. We had spent the full day there, and I was ready for going back to the resort. It was almost midnight, and the boys were still on one of the rides after queuing for over an hour, which seems to be the case for just about all the rides.

'Shall me and you walk steadily back to the car Dad, while Geoff stays with the boys?' Margaret suggested, 'they can catch us up if we take it steady. They shouldn't be too long.'

We had left my wheelchair behind at the chalet; as we knew we would be able hire one at the resort. Jaysus, we were soon to regret that decision. As Margaret and I worked our way back to the car, we dropped the wheelchair off at the reception area before stepping outside of the theme park. The place looked so different to how it had looked in the morning. Everything was lit up like Las Vegas, with dazzling lights and big buildings which we never noticed on the way in. I'm sure Margaret was thinking the same as me, because she looked over her shoulder towards the main gate with a concerned look on her face. When we had arrived in the morning, we parked in a car park we thought was near to the theme park. However, we soon realised our journey was just beginning. We had walked for what seemed miles before standing on a walking pavement that travelled towards the park entrance; followed by another long walk down towards the entrance where the wheelchair service was. I suppose in the excitement of it all, we had forgotten about the walk back being just as far.

We had to retrace our footsteps uphill without a wheelchair. I was already weak and in a great deal of pain around my stomach and bladder area. I had tried to pass water before we left the park, but still felt as if I hadn't emptied my bladder. Walking towards the left hand side of the park, thinking that was where the car was, we soon realised we are going the wrong way. We were lost, and there was no point in going back inside the theme park. The place being so huge meant there was a chance we could miss Geoff and the boys. They were going to follow us after ten minutes or so and wouldn't be there. There was no choice but to try and find the car and the hill was much steeper than we had realised. It felt like my legs were giving way. I held on to my walking stick and Margaret's arm, looking for a place to sit down for a while. Eventually, we spotted a tree with a wooden seat around it. Realising we were completely lost, Margaret stopped people to ask for help, but of course they all spoke French, or other foreign languages. She was very close to tears by this time and she was blaming herself for not waiting for Geoff.

'We were stupid not to bring our mobile phones with us.' She cried, dabbing her eyes with my handkerchief, 'I knew the boys had a phone each, but that's no good if we were to get separated like we have. I don't even know their phone numbers to ring them from a call box . . . if there is such a thing as a phone box around here. What an idiot I am, putting you through all this. I'm so sorry Dad.' She dried her eyes. 'Will you be all right if I go and look for them by myself? I'll keep popping back to make sure I don't go off course again. We need a wheelchair; I have to find a first aid place.'

She reluctantly left me sitting on the bench, and ran in every direction trying to find anyone who could speak English, coming back and checking on me all the while. No one appeared to speak English, even though there were literally thousands of people around us. We had been lost for over an hour by this time, and we knew Geoff and the boys would be back at the car worrying where we were. She sat down beside me with her head in her hands exhausted. Suddenly, the strangest thing happened. A young man and woman walked towards us.

'What's up love?' the young man asked in a broad Yorkshire accent.

Not only was he from Yorkshire, but he was from our own town of Barnsley. Margaret explained our situation, and his wife sat with me while her husband went with Margaret to find a first aid station, and hopefully borrow a wheelchair . . . though that wasn't really going to solve the problem of knowing where our car was. The young woman was very comforting and must have thought me rude, as I was in too much discomfort to speak.

Within a short time Margaret and the Barnsley lad came walking through the crowd with two policemen and two ambulance men. And as they walked, the uniformed men firmly lifted young children out of the way, and placed them to one side while they wheeled a chair through for me. At this precise moment, the boys appeared. Apparently, they had run all over the site trying to find us and were extremely breathless. A few minutes after they arrived, Geoff came running from another direction. He too was breathless and clearly distressed. The strange thing was . . . there were thousands of people walking up and down; some coming out of Disneyland and some going in to watch the fireworks display, or on their way to the hotels. Yet, neither Geoff nor the boys would have seen us if they hadn't been drawn to the sight of four tall uniformed men moving everyone out of the way. They would probably have run straight passed us, as we were hidden by the tree. I looked around, but the young man and his wife seem to have suddenly disappeared. They were gone before we had chance to thank them.

We were taken to a first aid room where the paramedics checked me out. They wanted to take me to a hospital in Paris, but Geoff convinced them it was all down to me having Parkinson's disease. He managed to persuade them I would be all right, but we still had the problem of where we had parked the car, and I didn't realise until that point that Geoff didn't know either. The man from the first aid station crammed us all into his car, which was exactly the same as ours, to drive us around the huge car parks to look for our vehicle. On arriving early in the morning, the car park hadn't been busy, but by this time, there were literally thousands of cars, buses and vans parked up. Each car park apparently had a cartoon name which we hadn't noticed when we arrived. Luckily Antony had.

'It was Whinny the Poo car park, I remember it now.'

'Don't be stupid Ant,' said Nick.

'It was.' Antony replied 'I saw 'Whinny the Poo.'

'Yeah, you're full of poo.'

'Shurrup Nick.'

'You shurrup. Whinny the Pooooo.'

'Shurrup.'

They'd started to argue, thumping each other on the arm and Margaret yelled at them to be quiet. The man driving said it was worth looking at this car park; well . . . we assumed that's what he said, as his English wasn't so good. Suddenly there was our car. We thanked the man who was not at all amused, and he drove off without so much as a wave or a goodbye. I imagine he thought we were all idiots.

The journey back to the chalet was a long way, and seemed longer still as the blackness enveloped us along the country lanes. Villages we passed through were still, and quiet without a soul, but then, it was the middle of the night. We arrived back to the chalet at three in the morning.

The next day Margaret started singing.

'I was lost in France
In the fields the birds were singing
I was lost in France
and the day was just beginning . . . '

Funny, how trauma can soon turn to laughter. We were talking about how fortunate it was that, out of all those thousands of foreign people, someone from Barnsley had come to our rescue. Margaret had the answer to that question.

'They were 'Earth Angels' sent down to help us. They walk among beings that need help. Why do you think they just disappeared? None of us saw them leave. Didn't you think that was strange? They appeared out of nowhere and disappeared into nowhere. Out of all those crowds of people, someone turned up from Barnsley. What was the chance of something like that happening? They were Earth Angels.'

Thank God for Earth Angels.

The day after the drama in Disneyland it poured down with rain, but it was still very warm and we travelled further afield, sightseeing, stopping off in various places to walk around. The boys hired canoes, making their way to the lake when we arrived back at the resort, and later in the evening we played games and cards, which was boring. Margaret shuffled the cards and started to 'read' them to Nick, doing a bit of fortune telling. It was all taken in fun and we laughed the rest of the night, it was better than playing cards and not taken seriously. I was very tired that night, and as soon as my head hit the pillow, it wasn't long before I fell into a deep sleep.

I was suddenly woken by a man in a black gown with a hood covering his head and face. He told me Margaret was in danger and I had to save her.

'You have to save her from evil. I am an Earth Angel sent to help. We have to save her Patrick.'

Three times he said this before drifting away into the wall. I got out of bed and dressed myself as quickly as possible, struggling with each of the buttons on my shirt. I had a problem getting my socks on my feet, the bed being so high, and I fell off three times before deciding to sit on the floor and do it that way. I tiptoed quietly without turning on the lights, and stood over the bed where they were sleeping. I started to say the Lord's Prayer and made the sign of the cross above Margaret's head, when she suddenly woke up.

'Dad what are you doing, it's the middle of the night . . . and why are you dressed?' Margaret yelled, trying to adjust her eyes to the darkness. Geoff woke up wondering what was happening. He jumped out of bed and gently guided me back to my room.

'Paddy, come on back to bed, you've been dreaming. You must have got a bit overtired. It was a long day yesterday and a bit traumatic to say the least. I'll help you undress and get you a glass of milk.'

I suppose Margaret mentioning Earth Angels had been on my mind when I went to sleep. Not to mention her 'reading' the cards. I must have scared the life out of them. They must have thought I'd gone mad standing over Margaret and praying. We laughed about it the following morning, but what an experience to go through. I had a few more nightmares while I was on holiday, and Margaret believed it was probably because I was out of my comfort zone.

*

It was soon time to go home and I dreaded the thought of all the travelling we had to do; but the journey to the ferry wasn't as bad as I'd thought it would have been. Travelling through the day, rather than the night made all the difference I suppose. We stopped a couple of times to stretch our legs before reaching Calais, and once on the boat I managed to walk around the deck and see the white cliffs of Dover coming into view. I slept most of the way home, waking only to get out of the car for something to eat, and walk around to stretch my legs again. I had enjoyed my first holiday abroad. For years I had thought how good it would be to visit the war graves and see places I'd only ever seen on television. I'm eighty years old now, and think how blessed I am to have fulfilled one of my dreams. Not many people get to visit a foreign country at my age. Not a beach holiday, but one of great adventure. Unfortunately, I didn't think much to Disneyland, but then I am rather old for that kind of thing. The boys said it had been the best holiday they had ever had and they've been abroad quite a lot. It was midnight when we arrived home and we were all eager to see our beds, I know I certainly was.

Now I had something else to add to my long term memory.

During the holiday I hadn't mentioned to Margaret and Geoff about the sores on my chest and stomach. I seemed to sweat such a lot, and the sores had started to leak. When I told Geoff he was shocked to see the open sores and immediately put cream on them.

'You might be better sleeping in just a cotton vest and boxer shorts, instead of pyjamas Paddy. I'll ring the surgery tomorrow and make an appointment. You might need antibiotics. They look very sore.'

I tried to sleep, putting nice thoughts into my head. Margaret had suggested doing this for preventing nightmares; but it wasn't helping. I dreamt someone was chasing me to get inside my body and take over my mind. I fought them off, but they came back again.

'What?' I yelled, 'What do you want from me? Leave me alone.'

Margaret came rushing into the room, and tried to reassure me it was just a dream.

'I'll get you a clean vest, the one you're wearing is wet through with sweat, and I'll change the pillow slips. Do you want a glass of milk or a cup of tea?'

'No, I'll be all right. I heard voices.'

'It was a bad dream Dad. I heard you shout. I'll sort you a vest and clean pillow slips out and then you might sleep better. It's three in the morning.'

New things were happening to my body, as well as my left leg swinging over my other leg; I felt dizzy and lost my balance just about every day. I had waited six months for my appointment with the specialist to take a look at my medication again, and he had given me a new tablet as well as the ones I was already taking. At first they seemed all right, but the downside was, I was always sleeping. I seem to fall asleep an hour after getting dressed. In fact I slept more hours than I was awake!

The dreams were still with me, and I saw shadows just out of the corner of my eye. I felt confused and very unhappy. Unfortunately, things were getting worse each day. I would walk from one room to another, and my body would freeze, meaning I couldn't move for a minute or two. I felt restless and fidgety when resting, and always wanted to stand up and walk. I heard voices in my head and wondered if I was suffering from dementia. Even my hair was suffering; large flakes of dandruff clung to my scalp. There was scurf stuck to my hair and I couldn't get a comb through it. That was the only time I had ever been grateful for not having a full head of hair. I mentioned it to Margaret and she looked it up on the computer.

'It appears to be Seborrhoeic Dermatitis. It says here, it happens a lot to people with Parkinson's disease. I'll see if we can get shampoo from the chemist and give it a go.'

The shampoo did manage to clear the dandruff up, but it needed doing regularly and Margaret spent ages combing out the bits that had stuck to my hair.

*

I can see the path that leads to the front door from where I sit, and they're coming. I know it's them. I knew they would come for me. I climb out of my chair and walk as quickly as my legs will take me upstairs, feeling as if I'm walking through a force which is holding me back . . . but I must get there. I literally pull myself up by the banister, and my body is heavy, my hands are sweating and my head is banging. But I have to hide because they're coming for me. I struggle to fasten my coat, my hands are stiff and I can't grasp the zip. I hear voices downstairs. Perhaps if I slip out of the back door . . . but then they will be waiting at both doors, and what if Margaret lets them in before I can get downstairs. I pace the floor wondering what to do. I hear a shout from Margaret. Keeping perfectly still, I stay where I am, confused and frightened.

'Dad, where are you? What are you doing up there? Christopher has just arrived.'

I stay quiet and Margaret rushes upstairs.

'What's the matter Dad? You look like you've seen a ghost, are you feeling all right? Are you coming down? Christopher is here.'

'Christopher', I reply, shocked to say the least. 'I thought I saw the police walking up the path, come to arrest me about those kids.'

'It's not the police Dad, its Christopher, and what kids are you talking about? You've got yourself into a right state. You were reading the paper this morning about those paedophiles being arrested. You must have had a nightmare about it all . . . and you did actually fall asleep whilst reading the paper. It must be something to do with the Levo-dopa tablets. The doctor said they could cause hallucinations.'

She reassuringly put her arms around me and guided me to the stairs. 'Come on down now and I'll make you a cup of tea.'

Now I have delusions and hallucinations. What next?

We walk downstairs and Margaret is still trying to set my mind at rest, saying it was a dream. I'm shaking all over . . . not from Parkinson's, which has almost stopped since taking the new tablets, but from fear.

Margaret hands me a cup of tea and tries to calm me down. 'You're new to these tablets and they will take some getting used to. If this continues, I'll phone the Parkinson's clinic and try to make an earlier appointment, but we have to give them a try first.'

She showed me the newspaper article I had read, and suggested it would be best to avoid looking at articles like this for the time being. She also said it would be a very good idea not to watch anything violent, or disturbing on the television. Handing me a cup of tea, my hands still shaking, she said to me.

'If I watch anything violent, I have nightmares myself. I hate those types of films anyway, and avoid them. Really, you could do with watching funny films to make your facial muscles work better. I remember you always did like a good laugh, and laughing is supposed to keep you young looking you know. There's a channel on Sky television which has all your old favourites on, such as 'Last of the Summer Wine' and 'Fawlty Towers.'

I did just that. I watched 'One Foot in the Grave' and laughed as I had done with Joyce the first time it was on the television. After that dreadful morning it was agreed I should avoid reading the news until we had seen the specialists to sort my medication out. I no longer watched anything on television that might have a negative effect on my mind either. I was not getting used to the medication. I saw spiders weaving webs and I waved my hand to people in the garden who, apparently, were not there. The hallucinations were making my life a misery.

On another occasion I called out, 'Margaret, there's two little girls coming up the path, one girl with black hair and one with ginger hair. They must be at the front door by now.'

She looked outside but no one was there, and I felt like I was going insane.

'Perhaps it's just an old memory of me and Teresa when we were young. Our minds can play funny tricks on us. Your description really does describe us both.' Margaret sat beside me and held my hand. 'Those tablets must be playing havoc with your mind. You're not going mad, you are perfectly sane, and you certainly don't have dementia. It's the medication that's causing you to see things that are not there. Your appointment isn't far away now. We'll have a word with the specialist about it all and see if he can change your tablets. He's a very good doctor and I'm sure he'll sort everything out. I suppose its all trial and error with everyone who has Parkinson's. It really does go to show everyone is different, and has completely different symptoms.'

She looked at the leaflets from the medication and sighed. 'It's not much of a life for you if you're sleeping all the time. Nor does it help with the terrible dreams you are having, they're so confusing for you, and it's got to the point where you don't know what's real anymore. There has to be something else you can take.'

True, I wasn't sure anymore what was real, or what was my imagination . . . or hallucinations, as they call them. Margaret was right. I was drifting off to sleep all day, and getting motivated was harder than ever, even getting up from a chair was a chore. We managed to laugh off the hallucinations as much as possible, which was helpful to me. They never laughed at me, but with me. For example, I was in the lounge, while Margaret was in the kitchen, when I saw my mother, who at the age of eighty nine, died in 1993.

'Who is it you're talking to this time?' she called out.

'My mother' I shouted back.

'Well then, tell her to bugger off, you're not ready for going over there yet. Tell her you'll see her in ten years time or so.

'Chapter Seven

Christmas in hospital

(2006)

'It's time to go back to the house now Bonny.' I said wearily. The dog looked up at me with a puzzled look on her face. We had only been in the field for ten minutes or so and I felt tired. Making my way back to the gate, I could see Margaret watching me from the window, and I guessed she'd probably been there since I had left the house. I was exhausted: four times I had woken up during the night to pass water, which isn't easy as it's a struggle to get out of bed, and I'm no sooner back in bed when I have to get up again. I have walked Bonny around the school fields at the back of the house almost every day since Margaret and Geoff came to live with me. Sometimes, we could be out for an hour stopping to talk to people and strolling along with them. I worked on those schools when we first moved into the house. There were four originally, but now, only two are left for the younger children. One of the senior schools has been demolished, and the remaining one has been turned into council offices. I still remember when the teachers and the school children planted Horse Chestnut trees in the playing fields over fifty years ago; now the leaves seem to whisper in the breeze as they rustle.

Margaret asks if I'm all right. She tries hard to let me keep my independence, but needs to watch me from the window in case I fall down, especially as my left foot is still swinging over to the right.

'I'm all right. I just feel really tired and sluggish, and sometimes it's too much of an effort to get out of my chair. I put it down to not being able to sleep right through the night, and having to wake up all the time for a pee.'

'I know you do, I hear you sometimes, and notice your bedroom light shining out onto the landing. I'm a bit concerned really. You're putting a lot of weight on around your stomach, and I've noticed you don't seem to be going to the toilet much during the day; you only went twice all day yesterday. Try drinking more water, and go to the toilet just to try and pee, even if you don't feel like going.'

I think that was more of an order than a suggestion, as every two hours or so, she would ask me if I ought to try and go. I do have difficulty passing water, my bladder always feels full, but I hardly ever pass anything during the day, even when I try.

Is this one of the so called symptoms of Parkinson's disease?

Margaret is like a Rottweiler when she has a hold of something. She won't let go. A few weeks went by and Margaret mentioned my problem again. 'I've noticed you don't walk Bonny around the field as much you used to. Are you in any pain or discomfort you're not telling me about Dad?'

'No. I'm all right.'

'You're not passing water during the day . . . not as much as you should be for the amount of tea you drink. You can tell me you know.'

'It's embarrassing.'

'People die from embarrassment. They hold on to things and then it's too late.'

'Well, it's not just having difficulty passing water, sometimes I have difficulty reaching the bathroom in time . . . and I dribble into my boxers.'

'I'll phone social services and ask if they can help. They might be able to give us some advice. Don't worry; they won't know who you are. The only other option is to make an appointment to see the doctor.'

'Try the social services first because they won't know who I am.'

The lady at the other end of the phone was very helpful, and gave Margaret a telephone number for someone who she said could arrange for us to pick up some pads for the leaks.

'I'm not wearing those.'

'It's nothing to be ashamed of; both men and women wear pads at some point in their lives, even young people.'

After much persuasion, realising the pads would be much better than wearing damp underclothes; I decided to give them a go. It must have taken me twenty minutes or more in the bathroom to work out how the sticky tape worked. Eventually, I pulled up my shorts and trousers and came out of the bathroom, only to find it felt like walking with a lopsided flannel between my legs. No one mentioned you needed to use Y front underpants. We went shopping for new underwear, and I have to say the pads did help with the leaks, but of course they made no difference to the fact that I still had trouble passing water during the day. I decided to tell Margaret.

'I'll phone the urology clinic and ask them what we should do. Though I suppose they'll say we have to see the doctor about it, and if so, then you'll have to go. It isn't anything to be embarrassed about Dad.'

'Well I suppose so'

I heard her telling someone on the other end of the line about my problem. She said "alright" and gave them our address.

'They're going to send someone out to do a bladder scan on you.'

'When are they coming?'

'Now . . . We need to get it seen to.'

How were they going to do that?

In less than an hour a man in a white coat arrived with some sort of machinery. Margaret left the room and I'd started to undress.

'You don't need to take anything off, just unzip your trousers so I can scan your bladder, Mr Millar.'

There was no pain or needles and it didn't take long at all. When Margaret came back into the room, the man in the white coat informed both of us that he needed to immediately insert a catheter into my bladder.

'His bladder is dangerously full,' he said with concern 'and could flow back up into his kidneys. It needs doing now.'

'Insert a catheter?' Margaret was shocked. 'Does he really need a catheter? Will he have to have one permanently if you do that? I'll have to have a word with my own doctor first to see what he suggests. He might give him some tablets for it.'

The man argued with her that it should be done straight away, and Margaret eventually gave in.

The feeling of relief was unbelievably good.

Follow up appointments were made to see an Urologist at the hospital, and I was told I needed a catheter on a permanent basis. I was shocked to find I had to have a bag strapped to my leg twenty four hours a day. Almost immediately, I started having pain and soreness, and as the weeks went by, urine infections seemed to be a regular occurrence. Right from the onset of being fitted with a catheter I suffered pain in my lower stomach area and in my back, and I always seemed to be on antibiotics.

It was arranged for me to have an investigation at the hospital to rule out anything serious. The procedure was painful and left me very sore. It was carried out in theatre, and I suppose I had to be grateful when the surgeon said it wasn't cancer. Pleased as I was about the news, it wasn't going to take away the pain or discomfort of having a tube attached to my privates. Within a matter of weeks, after having the investigation, I started with another infection, and this one affected my brain. I have no memory at all of the day when it happened, but this is what I was told.

That particular morning I was having my breakfast in the conservatory, because the kitchen and dining area were full of the furniture from the front room, as a new carpet was being fitted later in the day. Margaret was surprised when she entered the conservatory to find me staring into space, with a spoon sticking

94

out of my mouth. She laughed at first, thinking I was being funny, but became increasingly worried when I started to giggle in a strange way. Apparently, I took the spoon out and told her that I was born with a spoon in my mouth. She fed the rest of my breakfast to me and assumed I was tired. Ten minutes later she brought me a cup of tea, and I asked her if she knew my nurse.

'Dad, do you know where you are.'

'I'm in Kendray hospital.'

'What year is it?'

'1956. Why, don't you know what year it is?'

I had been admitted to Kendray hospital with pneumonia in the 1950s. Pneumonia was a killer at the time and I had almost died. My mind had gone back to the days I spent there. I was incoherent and said silly things, so Margaret phoned the doctor and cancelled her client's appointments.

Margaret told me later it was one of the strangest days she'd ever had. As well as the new carpet being fitted, we were having cable television installed on the same day. The doctor's receptionist said it would be after lunch before a doctor could come out to see me, so Margaret sat me in the reclining chair, and as I was shivering covered me with a blanket. Teresa came by taxi, but on arriving she ran straight to the toilet to be sick. Margaret said Teresa looked very ill and insisted on phoning her doctor to arrange to take her there; and was booked in for an early afternoon slot. I was getting worse as the morning went on, becoming very delirious, and according to Margaret I was losing quite a lot of blood in my urine. Margaret panicked and instead of waiting for the doctor, she called an ambulance.

The man came to fit the cable television just as the ambulance arrived, so she left the job of signing for it to Teresa, who by this time looked like 'death warmed up' as Margaret put it. Margaret came to the hospital with me in the ambulance, and sat with me for a few minutes, before going home by taxi to pick up the car to take Teresa to her doctor's surgery. Just as well, because Teresa had accidently been overdosing with the medication she was taking at the time. Margaret had to take Teresa home after seeing her GP, and then return to the hospital to bring my tablets and the other things I needed. After spending a short time with me at the hospital, she had to rush home for the carpet man. To her relief, Geoff arrived as she was leaving. Once again I was in the casualty department for seven hours before being admitted to a ward.

I do remember some of the time I was in hospital, but not much. They told me later that when Tony came to see me I was shouting out loudly and chuckling all the time, and I didn't recognise him. Margaret came back to the hospital with Geoff and was very upset because I didn't know who they were either. I was saying silly things which made no sense. The nurse assured them it was a urine infection, and explained how it can sometimes have an effect on the brain, leaving a sufferer confused. The next day Teresa, Kevin and Patrick came to see me and I was fine. From Margaret and Tony's description of the previous day, it was hard for them to believe how disorientated I had been.

I wasn't in hospital long before being allowed home, but while I was in there I made friends with the man in the next bed. He too was having problems with water infections, but he didn't have friends or family to sit with him. When the doctors came around to check on us, one of them very firmly told him to drink plenty of water. The poor man was weak, and was lying flat out on his bed with an intravenous drip in his arm. His water container and glass were placed on his meal trolley, at the far end of his bed, and I tried to shout.

'Yeah, well he would drink plenty, if he could reach the bloody water.'

*

I had enjoyed myself at the rehabilitation classes so much, meeting new people and all the laughs we had on those days, so through Social Services, Margaret and Geoff arranged for me to go into respite once a week. They thought the change would be good for me, and give them time to do things on their own. Instantly, I had a picture in my mind of it being something similar to the rehabilitation.

'What do you think Dad? Are you going to give it a go? It's entirely up to you.

'Yeah, I'll give it a go.'

When the transport bus arrived, Margaret stood at the door to wave me off. I couldn't help but feel sad knowing our roles had changed. She was the parent, and I was the child going to school on my own for the first time. A lump came to my throat. This was also the first time I had been anywhere on my own since having a catheter fitted, and I was nervous. It seemed to take forever to get there; with all the people we had to pick up on the way. No one glanced at me, nor did they look happy to be going to the day-care centre. This concerned me greatly. We were shown to a lounge where we all sat in a semi circle; I suppose to be able to speak to each other . . . not that anyone spoke, nor did they answer when I asked a question.

In all my life I can't remember seeing as much misery in a group.

A member of staff made us a cup of tea, but within an hour most of the group were asleep in their chairs. This was not at all what I had expected, and was completely different to the exercise classes I had been to at the hospital. Apart from a radio in the background, and the sound of someone vacuuming, there was a kind of unwelcome silence.

I found it hard to believe I was sitting amongst old folk in an old folk's home. I had always considered myself young at heart, and not ready for this kind of life. I read the paper again and again . . . well I pretended to; I had no interest in reading, I couldn't concentrate. When lunch time arrived, a carer came to take us to the dining room, and we ate our meal without a hint of enjoyment. A few of the permanent residents talked amongst themselves a little, but they still had a look of discontentment. I sat at the table after lunch thinking of Joyce, and how she would have hated being in a place like this. Eventually, we were steered back to the lounge like sheep. Within a short space of time, most of the group were asleep again.

Later in the day my catheter bag was emptied. Not in privacy, but in front of the rest of the group and I was embarrassed. One poor woman went into the toilet and came out leaving a trail of excrement, which was all down her legs, and I didn't know where to look. My heart went out to the woman, who appeared to be oblivious to it.

Another woman, sitting opposite me, had her legs open wide showing her big pink bloomers. Not a pretty sight.

Please dear God, let me die rather than spend the rest of my life like this.

I could hear one of the staff shouting at a resident, and the poor man came out of his room crying and wiping his eyes, followed by a young carer.

Old age will come you one day young lady and you may find yourself in a place like this.

When I finally arrived home, Margaret asked if I had enjoyed my day out.

'Yes, it was great', I lied.

It was only one day a week after all. Geoff was self employed, and to help Margaret, had decided to cut his days down to three days a week. They would be able to have a day out by themselves when I was in the day care centre, and this would mean Margaret would get a break from working and running around after me.

However, the same evening Geoff noticed I was very stiff when he helped me to undress, and commented that I must not have moved around much in the nursing home. Both Margaret and Geoff try to make sure I move around during the day to prevent me from getting stiff, and it was true what he had said, I didn't move much at all in the day care centre. I spent the rest of the week thinking about having to go back there again, until the day finally arrived.

My heart sank, as once again we all sat back down in a circle with a cup of tea in our hand. Fortunately for me, the week before I had left my new coat behind, and this meant I needed to wear a different coat to travel in. Margaret was concerned I would forget to bring both coats back with me and that one might get lost. The nursing home wasn't very far away, so a couple of hours after I'd arrived she decided to pick the coat up herself. I was surprised to see her when she turned up just like that, out of the blue. She walked towards me and saw me sitting in a chair reading the paper while most of the group were asleep. Margaret looked around the room and back to me again.

'Dad, are you OK? Where is everyone, and why are you sat around people sleeping. What the hell do you do here all day?'

I told her we read the paper and listened to the radio. I felt like crying by this time and wanted to go home. Thankfully Margaret sensed my sadness.

'Come on, get your coat, you might as well sit and read at home. You're not staying here.'

The care home assistant wasn't very happy about Margaret deciding to take me straight home, and later, the lady from Social Services said I shouldn't have just stopped going, but I was so relieved not to be going there again. However, a while later they were speaking to someone else from Social Services, who told them about a good respite home, that was nearby. She told them how it had a conservatory overlooking a nice park, but I didn't want to go to another nursing home, I would feel very old there. I wanted to stay in my own home. The problem was that I couldn't say too much when they made arrangements for me to go, and so I went along with it.

The morning for me to go on respite soon arrived, and as it was quite near to where we live, instead of me going on the transport bus, Geoff decided to take me and bring me back himself. When we arrived I climbed out of the car, feeling very emotional. I was never the sort of person to cry in front of anyone before I had Parkinson's disease, but the nursing home did appear to be very nice, and the staff seemed friendly enough, so I tried to cheer up.

Geoff walked in with me and handed my medication to the lady in charge. I felt happier to stay in this home and would give it a try, even if I didn't like it. I wasn't going to complain. Margaret and Geoff have a life too.

The day dragged by, just as it had in the last home. I was still surrounded by people snoring, but the views were much nicer from the large windows, and there were a few people who liked to talk this time. An hour or so after lunch I started to feel strange. My arm began to tremble, something that didn't happen since taking my new medication, and my insides started shaking. My whole being was jerking and I couldn't keep still. It was embarrassing. My head was falling forward, and I was heavy and stiff.

What the hell was happening to me?

Finally, Geoff arrived to pick me up, and the nurse returned my medication boxes. He had just put one day's supply of tablets in the boxes so he knew straight away they had missed giving me my tablets. I could see he was very annoyed about this, but managed to keep calm, considering I was given my tablets on the dot at home. Geoff explained to the nurse about the importance of giving me my medication precisely as directed on the boxes, and how vital it was not to miss a dose. Pointing to the medication, he stressed how missing a dose, or the tablet not being given at the correct time, could have a lasting effect on the whole day. The nurse apologised and said she would look into who had been responsible for giving medication out that day, assuring him it wouldn't happen again.

The following week, on my second visit, they missed giving me my tablets again and the same thing happened. I became jerky and shaky and felt strange as if there was an alien inside of me. This time Geoff was fuming with the staff and threatened to report them, which he eventually did.

That was the end of respite days and good riddance to them.

*

The urine infection returned a few months later, and I was sent to the day ward again for further investigations. This time, they were going to look deep inside to see if there was an underlying problem. I was wheeled once more down to the theatre in my green gown, ready to go through the procedure, and after what was a thorough examination the surgeon reported that there was nothing sinister going on.

Sinister, does he mean as in evil, menacing, or creepy?

He continued to tell me the cause of the infections was due to my having a long term catheter, and how very common it was to contract frequent infections, suggesting that the catheter was emptied as little as possible. Once again, we were never given any advice on this matter, and Margaret was concerned she might have caused the infections herself by emptying my bag too often. She had thought it would be easier on my leg, if it was an empty bag rather than a full one. We took his advice, but, unfortunately, this did not stop the infections from re-occurring, and they were becoming much more frequent. Not very long after the investigation procedure, yet again I was rushed into hospital in the middle of the night and this time I was really ill.

Is this how my life is going to be from now on? Am I going to have one infection after another, just as soon as the antibiotics have worn off?

I had been taken by ambulance to the hospital where the accident and emergency doctor changed my catheter to examine me. It had only been changed by the district nurse a few days earlier, so this was the second time in a week. Each change is a very painful procedure, and there is a greater risk of infection being introduced every time it's done.

Once again after lying in an uncomfortable position for six hours, waiting for a bed, my heels and bottom had become painful from lying on the trolley. I was also having trouble with my neck. Since first being diagnosed with Parkinson's I had been unable to straighten my spine, and although the bed was raised to a sitting position, I had been unable to relax my head for all those hours. Margaret had asked a nurse for a pillow but was told they don't have pillows in the casualty department. She removed her coat to tuck under my head, but this didn't help much. When I was finally admitted to the ward, I was only given one pillow, which didn't support my neck sufficiently. When we asked for extra pillows, the nurse had said there were none available.

When the junior doctor arrived to assess me, he asked questions I didn't fully understand, and the less I understood, the louder his voice became.

Why do some doctor's automatically assume you're deaf when you're older? I'm neither deaf nor daft. I just didn't understand the questions.

Much to Margaret's horror, the doctor was about to change my catheter again.

'Excuse me', she said very loudly, 'he had a catheter change downstairs in casualty only a couple of hours ago, and he had his regular change earlier in the week, not to mention having an investigation only a few weeks ago in theatre. Why are you doing one again?'

'Because I'm a doctor and I need to examine him. I want to see for myself. Is that all right?'

'But they're painful procedures and . . .'

'Excuse me. Do you mind? Can I get on with my job?'

He spoke in a very abrupt way, and for a moment I thought Margaret was going to say something else, but she had decided against it.

As the hours wore on I had become extremely ill, and in the middle of the afternoon visiting session I projectile vomited all over my son Patrick, hitting him full force as he walked towards my bed. I was shaking violently and thrashing around, while the doctor and a nurse tried to hold me still. They started to shout loudly, as if I was deaf, telling me to calm down while they examined me. Margaret was shouting at them to stop.

'He's having a panic attack. We see this all the time when he has a water infection, and panic attacks are also part of the symptoms of Parkinson's disease if they become distressed. Leave him alone and he'll be all right in a few minutes. Let me talk to him. You're frightening him.'

They carried on and ignored her pleas and she rushed out of the ward, telling me she was going to phone Geoff. The hospital is just a short distance from home and within twenty minutes, Geoff arrived, but the doctor had gone, and so had my panic attack. Geoff asked me if I was all right and looked at my chart. He was shocked to see they hadn't given me any Parkinson's medication. Including being in casualty, I had been in hospital almost a full day by then, and no one had given me my medication. Geoff was not happy about this and asked to speak to the doctor.

'No wonder my father-in-law had a panic attack, he hasn't had his Parkinson's medication since ten o clock last night. He left home in the early hours of this morning and they were brought with him. We always give him his medication on time, it's very important to give the correct dose at the same time every day.'

This appeared to have fallen on deaf ears, and there was a heated argument, as the doctor explained that medication is given out to patients at certain times of the day. He continued to state.

'We're going to change his medication and this takes time.'

Margaret was fuming, and spoke before Geoff had the chance to.

'Why are you changing his medication? That episode was to do with his water infection. I keep telling you, we see this all the time when he has a water infection. He's been settled on this medication since his Parkinson's consultant put him on these tablets. There are only a few side effects and he's settled down with them now. It's taken a long time to get it right. You need to contact his Parkinson's specialist before you change his medication.'

The doctor stopped what he was doing and looked at Margaret.

'I'm sorry, but are you a doctor?'

'No, I'm not a doctor. Are you a Parkinson's specialist?'

Margaret stormed out of the ward leaving Geoff with the doctor. There was more heated debate over changing my medication, but the doctor still did it his way, which, eventually, was to lead to serious consequences.

I had been admitted to hospital over a week ago, and because I was so poorly, I didn't realise how close it was to Christmas. The day before Christmas Eve, the ward consultant asked if I would like to spend Christmas at home with my family. Of course I said yes, even though I felt very ill.

Was he sending me home to die?

Geoff agreed to take me home providing they would let me back onto the ward, should anything happen for the worse. This would prevent another long wait in casualty, as my previous six hour wait had caused pressure sores on my heels and bottom. The consultant agreed and said it wasn't a problem. I distinctly remember Geoff asking him a few times to verify, if I was taken ill once I was home, I wouldn't have to spend hours on end on a hospital trolley. Each time the consultant said I could come straight back to the ward.

I was home for less than an hour when I wanted to go to the toilet to open my bowels. As I tried to stand, I crumpled to the floor in agony, shaking violently and my muscles went into a spasm. Geoff and Tony had great difficulty getting me back onto a chair. Apparently, my temperature was sky high, and I was obviously still suffering from the water infection. Geoff phoned for an ambulance, explaining I was to go straight back on the ward.

I was taken straight to casualty.

We arrived in casualty and I was put on a trolley in a side ward, once again without a pillow. Geoff spoke to a doctor who came to see me, explaining how I had only been home for an hour and shouldn't be in casualty.

'The consultant on the ward said my father-in-law could go straight back up to the ward if his condition worsened. He'd only been home an hour. He was in casualty for six hours last time, even longer the time before. He has bed sores on his heels and buttocks, which he didn't have before he came in here. He's in a lot of pain. It's as if everyone has just given up on him.'

The doctor didn't really say much other than it's not their policy for a patient to go straight to a ward without being assessed by a doctor first. He wasn't very sympathetic, and couldn't say how long I would be this time. Geoff was angry.

'They had no intention of letting him go back to the ward. We were tricked into my father-in-law being allowed home, just so they could get as many patients as possible out for Christmas. Not for the patient's sake, but for theirs.'

I was in casualty for another six hours

I started to go downhill from then on. The infection didn't clear up, in fact, it worsened and I was feeling strange again. At first I didn't know where I was, and I was told later I had slept for most of the time. I was aware of food being left for me, but being too weak, I couldn't feed myself and the food was taken away. The glass of water was out of my reach, and the only time I was able to drink, was when my family came to visit.

Eventually, the infection was starting to ease and I was allowed to sit in a chair at the side of the bed. My feet were freezing on the cold floor, and I was plagued with terrible sores on my heels and bottom. Of course, being in casualty for the second time had only fuelled the problem. I was unable to wear slippers or socks because of the pain, and I was either in bed or in the chair for hours at time. I hadn't walked, or stood up for over a week and my bottom was starting to get so painful that I wanted to scream out loud, shifting my bottom from one side to another, in the hope it would take the pressure off. Just over a couple of weeks ago, I was walking around the house and garden using my walking stick. Now I wasn't able to walk. I was also constipated. I couldn't relax enough to open my bowels sitting on a commode with people around me, even though the curtains were closed. It's very embarrassing. The days dragged on and the pain was far worse. Margaret sneaked in before visiting, and saw me wince when I moved.

'It can't be good for you sitting on your bum all day Dad, you'll get trapped wind. Have you been to the loo since you came into hospital?'

I told her I hadn't and that I had stomach cramps. She went quiet for a while and . . .

'I know this might sound crude Dad, but you need to stand up and have a good fart.'

I laughed; it's something we never do at home, not in front of anyone, but she wasn't joking.

'Come on Dad, stand up and let that wind out. There are only three patients in the ward, and it's not visiting time yet. Passing wind is a natural bodily function. They can like it or lump it. You haven't been to the loo for over a week, and it might help if you pass wind. Remember that old saying. "Where ere you be, let the wind go free, in church or chapel, let the buggers rattle.' She laughed. 'Seriously Dad, you must be full of painful wind.'

I stood up holding on to her arm and let the wind out. I couldn't believe I was doing this, not just for other people to hear, but in front of my own daughter. I bet you could have heard the sound across town. It rattled and blew for quite some time, and luckily the other three patients in the room thought it was funny.

'Jaysus, I feel much better now.'

I certainly did, but I really needed to open my bowels even more now.

All the family came to visit, and the nurses kept moaning about extra visitors at my bedside. I was only supposed to have two visitors at a time, but I have five kids who are all concerned about me, and then there was Geoff. I couldn't remember how long it had been since I last went to the toilet to open my bowels. Laxatives didn't work, and finally Margaret asked if I could be wheeled to the toilet on a commode to go in private. Tony asked the nurse if he could wheel me to the toilet himself, but she insisted on taking me herself, leaving me on the commode and telling me to pull a cord when I was finished. Thank God, I managed to open my bowels; all I needed was a bit of privacy. I waited for the nurse, but soon realised she must have forgotten me. The toilet door had been left slightly open, so I tried to stand and make my way back to my bed. Unfortunately I fell forward, banging my head, elbows and

106

thigh. My voice was too weak to shout for a nurse, and I seemed to be there a long time before I heard Margaret and Tony talking outside. They had come looking for me because I had been some time, assuming the nurse was in with me. With all my strength I shouted as loud as my lungs would allow. Margaret and Tony came rushing in to help me. They pulled the emergency cord, but it was still quite a while before a nurse came. Tony asked the nurse why she had left me on my own when I hadn't been able to stand up without support. The nurse said she was busy with another patient and didn't have time to wait.

'I left him on the commode and told him to pull the cord.' She argued. To which Margaret replied.

'I can't believe this, my dad doesn't know a 'cord', he has a bad water infection, and his mind isn't working properly. Why didn't you let my brother go with him in the first place?'

The nurse apologised and explained it was hospital policy for a nurse to escort patients everywhere, and that she had been called away to another patient. I was wheeled back to bed and I said to Margaret and Tony.

'I kept shouting for you but you didn't hear me. I thought I was going to be there all night.'

They asked to see the sister in charge, and explained how annoyed they were at my being left alone when I was clearly not myself.

'And another thing while we're at it,' Margaret said, 'they're taking my dad's food away before he has chance to eat it, and he isn't being given any water to drink only when we're here. He's lost a lot of weight since he came in here.'

Geoff arrived at that moment, but Margaret continued.

'Plus, he isn't being moved to take the pressure of the sores on his bottom. He's put on his bedside chair, where he sits for anything up to ten hours making matters worse. He's in pain from those sores.'

The discussion went on and Geoff mentioned to the ward sister about me having a 'Red Tray.' He had seen something about it on a poster downstairs. Having a red tray meant a nurse had to ensure you ate your meal, even feed you if necessary. Obviously the ward sister wasn't happy about this as they were short staffed. It was between Christmas and New Year, and in a way they were not to blame. Still my Red Tray was arranged.

Fortunately, because Margaret was having trouble lifting me from the falls I was having at home, Geoff was in the process of giving his job up to care for me. He was going to become my full time carer, and because of this, the sister gave him permission to come in at meal times and help me eat. He also persuaded the sister to let him come in the mornings to give me a shave. I hadn't had a shave for over a week, or a bath.

*

An official looking woman in a suit walked into the ward and towards me. She said she was going to take a water sample from my catheter, but she didn't say why. Margaret, who was visiting, moved to one side, curious as to why she wasn't a nurse. The lady told Margaret she had come to assess me prior to me being moved. As she clumsily emptied the liquid into a urine bottle, her hand slipped and the contents went all over the floor, and my feet. My feet were wet through. She rushed over to the sink to get some paper towels and began to mop the mess up. Margaret was horror-struck and dismayed.

'He has an infection in his bladder, I hope that's not going to cause a cross infection to the bed sores in his heel.'

But of course it did.

Opposite my bed was a man who I would say was about seventy, and had been transferred to the ward from casualty to recover from pneumonia. He was loud mouthed and a complete nuisance to the nurses and patients. He would often leave the curtains open while he stood there to relieve himself into his urine bottle; regardless of who was in the ward. Had I been well enough to shout, I would have told him to close the curtains, but that was taken out of my hands; he did it one day in front of Margaret. Standing at the end of his bed, facing forward and taking out his penis, he stood there and urinated into a urine bottle. Shocked, Margaret yelled.

'You dirty pig, why can't you shut the bloody curtains to do that.'

'Cos I don't want to, it doesn't bother me, why should it bother you?' he retorted.

Margaret jumped up from her chair and yelled back.

'As a matter of fact it does bother me. Do it again and I'll pour it over your bloody head.'

I have to say he drew the curtains after that, but the day after we saw a jug under his bed, it was one of the water jugs and it was almost full to the top with urine. She complained to the nurse who said she would sort it out. However, the jug was not removed until the cleaner came the following morning.

Did the cleaner wash the jug out and put it with the other jugs, or did she throw it away? Jaysus, I won't be drinking water again.

Chapter Eight

Rehabilitation

(2007)

The hospital decided I should go to a nursing home to recuperate. I think really, they wanted us out of the way. I just wanted to go home to my bed. I disliked being in hospital, I was always thinking of Joyce, and often thought I could hear her familiar footsteps coming down the corridor towards the ward. Eventually, a social worker came to pay me a visit. She informed me I would be going to a rehabilitation hospital to get my strength back before going home. She made it sound like a holiday camp. I wasn't convinced.

If it's that good why don't you go there then?

'The hospital has now done as much as they can for you, Patrick. You need specialist care and rehabilitation and . . .'

The woman carried on talking, but I was only half listening. I had heard of this so called rehabilitation hospital. They used to say when you went in there, you never came out again. It was well known that you were sent there when the hospital could do no more for you. In the old days, people went there when they had treatment for infectious diseases such as tuberculosis. Although, I have to say I haven't heard much about it these days, in fact, I thought it must have closed down.

'. . . and there's a nice lounge which families can use at visiting times, instead of sitting at the side of your bed. There are plenty of board games in the lounge, and there's usually a game of bingo a couple of times a week.'

She went on and on. I didn't want to go into another hospital. I wanted to go home.

Who the hell wants to play bingo or draughts in a rehabilitation hospital? How is that going to cure anything and how long were they expecting me to stay there?

When they moved me, Margaret and Teresa followed the ambulance in Margaret's car, and had to wait outside in the corridor while the doctors and nurses assessed me and took blood from my arm. The nurse also used a swab inside my mouth, up my nose and around my groin, but didn't say what for. My travel bag, which contained my pyjamas, underclothes, toiletries and towels had been placed at the bottom of the bed, and had there been any of my daytime clothes and shoes in the bag, I might have contemplated walking out. It wouldn't have been the first time. Years ago I once walked out of a hospital in Dublin. The doctors had drawn a line with a black pen on my abdomen, saying this was to be the place where, the following morning, they were going to cut me open to investigate a duodenal ulcer. I had been petrified at the idea and wearing the clothes I had gone into hospital with, I walked out with Joyce and the rest of the visitors. It was years before I finally succumbed to the operation.

Later that morning after I had been assessed, Margaret and Teresa were allowed into the ward, and I pleaded with my two daughters not to leave me there.

'Don't leave me here. Take me home with you,' I whispered. The room seemed deathly quiet compared to the last hospital. I looked around the ward and I could see five other people lying in bed. They all looked very poorly. 'People are brought here to die. Take me home.'

'Look Dad.' Margaret said firmly 'people are not here to die. I don't know where you get that idea from. They are all here to get well enough to go home. It's a myth about people not going home. I know at one time, when it was a sanatorium it may have seemed like that, but not anymore.'

I wasn't convinced.

'They used to come in with chest infections and they never came out again. 'I argued.

'It's true; people did come here with chest infections.' Margaret said; 'and it did use to be a tuberculosis sanatorium at one time, and people did die from TB. But that was years ago. This is a hospital for younger men and women, not just old people. Those days are gone Dad. Nowadays people recover from diseases that used to kill them. We have better drugs now, even better than Penicillin.'

'So why am I here then?'

'Because the doctors and nurses are more specialised in dealing with people who are recovering from a serious illness, and you still have a water infection that needs to be cleared up. You're not here to die, so don't be saying things like that.'

The three of us had sat in silence while we waited to see what was going to happen next and I thought about what Margaret had said about TB once being a killer. I remembered when I woke up in a morgue, or 'dead house' as it was known then. It was in the mid 1930s and I was only eight years old. At the time, every household in Dublin lost a child from one disease or another, particularly TB. In fact, I had many friends who died from TB in the overcrowded tenement houses. I remember whole families being wiped out. Diseases spread like wild fire in those days, and with as many as eighty people living in one tenement house, there were deaths all the time. I don't remember being admitted to hospital on the day they thought I had died, but I woke up in the 'dead house' with a sheet over my face. All around me stood trolleys with white sheets covering the bodies, and I don't remember anything after that. It was never discussed at any time, but I have a scar on my neck and I have no recollection of how it got there. When I grew up I asked my mother about the incident, but I could tell she was reluctant to talk about it, other than I'd been rushed to hospital where they thought I had died. Years later, Joyce told me it looked as if I'd had a tracheotomy at some point.

There seemed to be a lot more activity in this hospital, with nurses tending patients and running around doing one thing or

112

another. There certainly didn't seem to be a shortage of staff like there was in the last hospital. My daughters were only in the ward ten minutes before the nurse asked if they would wait back in the corridor. She had sat at the side of me and explained the tests had shown I had MRSA.

'What's MRSA' I replied.

'MRSA is a type of infection which is resistant to antibiotics.' I listened carefully as she told me MRSA infections are a particular problem in hospitals. 'Some people have MRSA on their skin or up their nose without it doing them any harm. However, these patients may develop infections if the MRSA spreads from the colonised skin area to an open wound, such as the one you have on your heel. We're going to have to move you to an isolation ward, Mr Millar.'

Very quickly after she had left the room, I was wheeled in my bed to a tiny room behind the nurses' station. I was surprised it wasn't a room with other patients who were in isolation, but a single room. Margaret and Teresa came in to sit with me, and I knew they were both upset over the news. We, like most people, didn't understand the MRSA bug, and had assumed you would die from the infection.

The room I was moved to was very small with, what I would call, an old folk's chair with a high back and wings at the side. There was a sink in the corner, a wardrobe, a chest of drawers and a television which stood on a small table. While there was a window overlooking a small grassy bank, I couldn't see anything of the corridor, or the nurse's station. One of the double doors to the room was closed and the other one was left slightly open. I heard people talking outside of the room and could just make out the end of a desk. The room was literally tucked away from the main wards, as far as I could tell, and I wasn't allowed to even go to the toilet, but told I had to use a commode in my room. When anyone entered the room, they had to wear a disposable gown and rubber gloves.

Leprosy!

Margaret and Teresa tried to reassure me it wouldn't be for long, and said I would be home in no time. Every day my family would come and visit and Geoff came in as often as possible to wash and shave me. The nurses were quite capable of shaving me, but I preferred Geoff to do it. He had been doing it for a while before I went into hospital and he was used to me sometimes jerking and being stiff. It took a bit of organising, but eventually the staff agreed that Geoff could come in just after breakfast. However, he had to leave and couldn't come back until visiting time. Time went by so quickly for me during visiting hours, but visiting times were very strict. The rest of the day dragged by, and I never spoke to a soul apart from a few nurses who took time to speak to me; they were all too busy. Doctors came and went, speaking to me as if I was deaf. Just like the other doctors had done, very loud, slow and precise.

'Now then Mr Millar, how are we today?'

I'd never come to grips with why a person would say, 'how are we.' I lay silent, as they spoke to each other as if I didn't exist . . . another thing all doctors do in hospitals, especially when they are training medical students.

I was feeling grumpy and angry, even though the members of staff were all extremely nice to me, and so were the doctors. One of the problems I was having was not being allowed to go to the toilet and having to use a commode. I wasn't even allowed to be by myself while I was sat on it. The two nurses who stayed with me used to chat to each other and look away, but it was still very embarrassing. I'd felt like a baby being placed on a potty. I told Margaret about my situation and she said the nurses were just doing their job. She said it was better than leaving me on my own, because I could fall and hurt myself again. I suppose she was right. The nurses did do their best not to make me feel uncomfortable, and I certainly couldn't complain about my being cared for. The hospital was kept spotlessly clean. My room was cleaned from floor to ceiling every day, and it was good having my room cleaned; I had someone to talk to, and the cleaners were very chatty.

The infection in my bladder was not yet responding to treatment, my Parkinson's medication was being looked into, but worst of all, was the pain in my heel. It had been dressed and put in, what the nurses called, a heavy dressing, which was a large padded boot that gave extra protection. The doctors were trying all kinds of different treatments on my foot, including silver and honey. The nurse told me one day, how silver was very effective for fighting infection, and I imagined my foot being wrapped in silver paper, but she told me the silver was impregnated into the dressing they were applying. Every Tuesday morning the nurses would wear a gown, mask and gloves to take a sample from my wounds. When the dressing was removed, I could tell from the nurse's face it had a bad smell, and I imagined it to smell of rotting flesh. I had no sense of smell anymore.

Another Parkinson's present.

Each and every day was the same. Weeks went by and I had no concept of time. I had no memory of Christmas at all. I was in the last hospital when Christmas had come and gone, but I had no recollection of any of it. Hours drifted into days and then the days merged into weeks, and all the time I was stuck in a small room. I still couldn't go down the corridor to the toilet and between the pain in my heel and the pain in my bottom; I never really got much respite. It was even difficult to sit comfortably in my old folk's winged back chair. I kept slipping forward and sliding off it, forcing me to use my arms to push against the chair and literally lift my bottom back into the seat. Geoff explained to me the physiotherapists put little blocks under the chair legs, to make the chair tip forward. It was so patients didn't sit in one position all the time, and end up getting pressure sores.

Eventually, the specialists changed my Parkinson's medication. I was prescribed a large red tablet that was difficult to swallow, and I had to take one four times a day. The nurse stood beside me and made sure I took my medication as they always did, but as soon as she left the room I would spit out the red tablet. From the start I had learned to hide it between my teeth and gums. The taste was vile, bitter and sticky. Sometimes the tablets would melt in my mouth while I waited patiently for the nurse to leave the room, and red dye dribbled down my chin onto my shirt. Margaret laughed one day at the amount of tomato soup she thought we had for lunch.

'You must have tomato soup everyday Dad. It's all over your fingers and down your front again. Shall I ask them to put a cover over you?'

A baby bib!

'No' I said quickly. 'I'll ask a nurse myself.'

She knew nothing about the new tablet, but one day during visiting time, I saw Margaret pick something up off the floor and turn it over in her hand to inspect it.

'Dad, what's this? It looks like a sweet or something. I haven't seen sweets like this before. It's too hard for a jelly bean. Do you know what it is?'

I shook my head and started to fidget with my handkerchief, but she wasn't going to let go.

'It could be a tablet, but I know it's not one of yours, you don't take red ones.'

'No, I don't take red tablets. The nurse must have dropped it.' I lied. I was happy enough to take the rest of the tablets, but the red one was difficult to swallow and got stuck in my throat.

The tablet had fallen on the floor earlier in the day, and it was out of my reach to pick up and hide. I couldn't so much as stand now, never mind walk with my rubber foot, so I had to find hiding places close to me. I hid a tablet in the tissue box and one in my sock. I had even hidden a few of them in my mashed potatoes when a nurse left the room for a few minutes. I was taking four of these tablets a day and finding somewhere to hide them was difficult. Somehow, I managed to put a few tablets right at the back of the drawers near the bed. I couldn't put them in the bin because the staff might have seen them, and anyway, it was too far out of my reach. Margaret became suspicious one day after Tony mentioned he had also found a red tablet, and she began to question me about it. I told her a nurse must have dropped some sweets, and I lied even further by saying she had offered me one. Margaret went out of the room to ask the nurse if I was on a red tablet, to which the nurse replied.

'Yes, a Stalevo.'

'Well he hasn't been taking them, and his Parkinson's is much worse this week I've noticed.'

The nurse was surprised and in defence told Margaret.

'I gave him the tablets myself; I know he takes them all. I stay and watch Patrick swallow them. We have to make sure all our patients swallow their medication.'

'Yes, but did you see him actually swallow the new one, the Stalevo. He's a very stubborn man, and if he doesn't want to do something, he will find a way out. I'm not blaming anyone, but I think he must be hiding the tablet in his mouth until you leave. It wouldn't be the first time.'

There must have been a meeting with the staff. I had to show them my tongue after my medication and they looked inside my gums too. I felt like a naughty boy, but then that's how I was acting, I suppose. I soon found out if I swallowed the tablet quickly enough, it didn't become too sticky and melt on my tongue. Suddenly, I felt really guilty. I could have got the nurses into serious trouble, and I vowed not to do something so silly again. One thing was certain. This hospital made sure I drank plenty of water, and that I ate my meals. They sat beside me, and even helped to cut the food into smaller pieces whenever necessary. They couldn't be more helpful.

*

The nightlights are switched on and it's deadly quiet, but I am awake. I was woken by a noise in my room. I catch a fleeting glance of a figure dressed in black which moved swiftly from one corner of the room to another. Another fleeting glance and I see him; he must be seven feet tall. Who is he? He's watching me. The room has gone cold and I feel a fear throughout my body. I thought the tales of the Shadow men weren't real . . . but they are real, and one is here. They wait for death . . . I'm going to die. I shout for the nurse.

'Are you all right Patrick?'

'There's someone in my room, over there in the corner.'

'No, there's no one there. Try to get some sleep. It's just a dream.'

Jaysus, I'm going back to being a child. Isn't that what I used to say to the kids?

I can't sleep. The Shadow man has left me restless. Out of all those ghostly tales I heard in Ireland, there were two things that frightened me and my cousins the most . . . the tales of the Shadow People and of course the Banshee. The stories of the shadow people, used to put the fear of God in me. The Nan used to say everyone has a shadow, but on a dark night some people can also see the shadow of a person who is dead. In my youth I often came home on a dark night, terrified to look at the shadow on the wall in case there were two. I try to sleep but my mind won't let me. I hear the Nan telling me about the Shadows.

"A dead person's shadow will follow you if you knew them in life, and that's why the shadow is cast in a different shape to your body. And then there are the demonic shadows. They are not human. Neither are they lost souls. The Shadow People will hide in a corner and watch you while you sleep. They are evil and aggressive and have been known to attack, and once here, they won't go away. Some say their eyes are like red rubies and others say they have no eyes. They are very tall and wear long cloaks and have hoods that cover their faces, or sometimes wear a large hat. The shadows are associated with bad luck or death, and will hang around a bedroom waiting for a person to die, moving swiftly from one corner of the room to another."

Time passed and I was feeling very depressed. I had convinced myself I was in a nursing home. Margaret and Geoff had promised they would never put me into a home; but had they? I was in pain with my foot, and I had open sores on my arm which needed dressing, from the fall in the last hospital. I had been told I also had

118

MRSA in my nostrils and bladder, as well as my arm and foot. I was trapped inside a tiny cell like room, and my body was riddled with one thing and another. I was desperately unhappy. I wanted to scream out.

I came into hospital with a common water infection. I could walk. Now I'm in a bloody wheelchair with a great big hole in my heel eating my foot away.

One evening when I was alone with Margaret I told her I'd had enough and wanted to die, and the only reason I was holding on was the thought of upsetting her, and the rest of the family.

'I can't live like this,' I cried out, trying to hold back the tears. 'It feels like I've been in here for years. There's no light at the end of the tunnel, it just goes on and on. Anyway, I was right when I said they come in here to die. I'm dying in any case aren't I? I just wish death would come sooner than later. They can't do any more for me; surely I should be getting better by now . . . but I'm not.'

'There is light at the end of the tunnel Dad. You're not dying. Don't be talking like that. The doctor warned you it would take time. You don't want to go home only to be brought back again. Do you?'

When the visitors had gone and I was alone again, I looked over towards the sink and saw miniature toy soldiers marching. One soldier fell down and the others marched around him until he stood up to join them. I was always seeing things. I saw faces in the wardrobe, and the Shadow man is still waiting for me, hiding in the corner of the room. He is real. He isn't my imagination. Eventually, I fell into a deep sleep.

Someone is tapping my shoulder. I look up and see Joyce, my mother, Molly, Tom and the Nan. It's a foggy day outside and I stand to look out of the window; I know someone special is coming to see me but I don't know who. The mist seems to be in the room now, but we're not in Ireland anymore, we're in England in front of a big coal fire. There's a special cosiness about this room, and I feel a warm glow inside. Joyce is smiling, and I'm suddenly aware of someone standing behind me. I turn, but I can't see who it is

119

through the mist. Everyone is looking at me now, waiting for my reaction. The mist clears and I am overwhelmed on seeing Uncle Jamie, and immediately give him a big hug. He's holding a big parcel in his hand.

'Hello Paddy. How are yea?'

I tell him about my foot and he hands me a parcel. I eagerly open it. It's a wooden leg.

'I don't need a wooden leg where I am Paddy. See, I have two legs now. I thought you might want to have it, just in case.'

'It's my foot that's infected Uncle Jamie; I don't need a wooden leg. I only need a foot.'

'You could always saw the foot off the leg Paddy.' Molly laughs.

My mother tells me not to worry; I won't need either a foot or a leg, because everything is going to be all right now. They are all so pleased to see me, and I thank Uncle Jamie for his kind thought, and for helping my mother to look after me as a child.

'Remember when you used to say your leg was cold even though you didn't have a leg there.' I say to him and he laughs.

The mist starts to drift back into the room, and I can't see them anymore. I feel the soft touch of Joyce's lips on mine, and beg her not to leave me again.

'Come back, don't leave me here' I shout loudly. I was fully awake by then and surprised to see a nurse standing over me, asking if I was all right. She handed me a tissue and said she would speak to the doctor first thing in the morning about my hallucinations, and dreams. I couldn't get the dream out of my head, and was convinced it wasn't really a dream, and that they had all come to see me. Uncle Jamie took the role of a father when I was a child, and I loved him. He died a short while after I left Ireland to come over to England at the age of twenty, and I was upset because I couldn't afford the passage home to his funeral. Uncle Jamie had lost his leg during the First World War and used to sit rubbing his empty trouser leg when there was nothing there, and often complained of his leg being cold.

The following day, the consultant tried to reassure me they were doing everything they could to find the right medication and dosage for my Parkinson's disease, but that it could take some time. I just prayed they would find a dose that didn't give me hallucinations, or send me into a zombie state, sleeping all day and having bad dreams.

I tried to escape a few times, falling down after only a few steps . . . I wasn't going anywhere with my rubber foot. I would sit on the high backed chair for hours, and the pressure from the chair still hurt the bed sores on my bottom. I had been given an air bed to sleep on, 'to help my bed sores,' so they said, but it kept me awake as it rippled up and down my body. At first, as each ripple moved slowly along the length of the bed, it felt as if someone was moving about underneath the mattress, and the humming sound of the electric pump would keep me awake all night. I did eventually get used to it. My bed sores weren't as painful, and the lull from the electric pump became a cosy sound. In time, I was really grateful for the air bed.

I often heard my family asking the staff about my progress, and they were told I had an infection in my bladder which was taking some clearing, as well as the problem with the MRSA. The doctors and staff never failed to listen to my family's questions about my condition, and they were completely honest and sympathetic with them. They were all very good, and I knew they were doing their best to make me well again. Unfortunately, I didn't share their enthusiasm. I was getting more depressed than ever and it was showing.

Tony came to see me, and said he had been speaking to Margaret. She had telephoned him to tell him I was depressed, and how I had talked of wanting to die. He was very upset to hear what I had told her. If I expected sympathy, I was wrong. Tony gave me a right earful about how Margaret and Geoff had cared for me all this time, and wanted me home as much as I wanted to go home. He praised the hospital doctors and staff, saying they were trying hard to get me well enough to leave the hospital. His face was red and serious as he said I was being selfish. When I tried to speak, he cut me off, and told me I should start to fight this thing and get better. With his palms held out he stressed:

'You won't get any better if you give up and feel sorry for yourself.' His voice softened a little, 'I know it's hard for you being in this room Dad, but it isn't permanent. You're not in a nursing home. I know that's what you think. You're in a very good rehabilitation hospital.'

We talked awhile and I promised him I would try hard to get well again and I realised I had been selfish.

*

Margaret had never been able to understand why my bed was tucked away in the corner, far away from a view of the corridor.

'If the bed was facing the door, along with your chair, you would be able to see out.'

'They might not let you do that.' I said to her.

'I don't see why not? It's not being able to see outside of the room that drives you mad, and makes you feel isolated. You can hear the nurses talking to each other, but you can't see anyone, which makes it even worse.'

'I know. I keep thinking someone is shouting out to me and I try to stand up.'

Margaret went to have a word with the nurses, who were all gathered around the nurses' station just outside my room. Looking back towards my room, they could see what she meant. From where they were standing, they would be able to see me and I would be able to see them.

The bed and chair were moved and so was the bedside table. It was good to see people again.

The afternoon of the next day, I heard a funny noise and was sure the bed was moving.

Oh my God, was this another of my hallucinations?

I was sinking into the mattress, and being sucked down, swallowed and squashed as the mattress enveloped me. I was sure this was not my imagination. This was real. I yelled, as loud as my voice would let me, for someone to come and help; but no one came. I was suddenly thrown on my side and pushed onto the rail at the side of the bed, my face pressed into the pillow. I felt as if I was being sucked out of this life, and at this point I realised I didn't want to die. I heard a sound, and twisted my head to look up. Margaret and Teresa were standing in the doorway, laughing so much I thought they had gone mad. Why weren't they helping me?

Was this a dream? Was I dreaming? Am I hallucinating?

It was neither a dream nor a hallucination. While I was sleeping, the cleaner accidently turned off the machine which controls the bed. The pump had stopped, so the bed had been gradually loosing air out of the mattress, and I was tossed from one side to the other. A nurse was called, and I was helped into my chair while the bed was put right. It was the first time I had laughed in months. It was real laughter. The talk with Tony had been good for me. I realised after he had gone home that no one had given up on me, not the doctors or my family. I had to start believing myself. I was in a hospital to be made well again . . . not an institution or nursing home. I felt happier and it was good to laugh. When we finally stopped laughing Margaret asked.

'Why didn't you ring the buzzer?'

'What buzzer?'

She held the remote in front of my face.

'This buzzer;'

'Oh, I thought that was the telly remote,' I smiled 'no wonder I couldn't get BBC One.'

'Dad, you're not daft, just stubborn, you knew what the buzzer was there for, but you just won't use it. The staff can't always hear you if you shout, that's why you have a buzzer. Anyway, changing the subject, me and Teresa have been into town and bought you this nice shirt and tie in lilac, your favourite colour. I'm going to hang it up here, on the back of the door to remind you this is the shirt you will be coming home in.'

The shirt was hanging on the door another month. I was not going home. I hated that shirt and I have never liked the colour lilac ever since.

They had found the correct dosage for my Parkinson's medication some weeks ago, but the real problems was the pressure sore on my heel, and the fact that I was still proving positive for MRSA. The good news was that I was allowed down the corridor in a wheelchair. For safety reasons, I could only go with my family at visiting times, and I had to be kept away from the other patients. Eventually, and after much persuasion from Geoff, there was talk of me going home, but not before the MRSA in my foot had started to respond to treatment. Unfortunately, the dressing was only changed on a Tuesday, so we had to wait yet another week for the test to come back from the lab. My family would keep asking the staff if the results had come back, time and time again.

The physiotherapists were trying to get me walking in readiness for my return home, but the pain in my heel was so great, I couldn't put the slightest pressure on it. Each day they came to the ward and spent about fifteen minutes working on exercises to strengthen my legs. My chair was still being altered by the physiotherapists; it was raised and tipped just as before, but now I was keen to use my arms to help build up my strength. They had brought me a special foam pad, about six inches deep, to put on the chair which was easier on my sores. Geoff told me the physiotherapists were really pleased with my progress and that he could help further by helping me to practice my exercises, and as much as we could, we went through the routines. I was really looking forward to going home and was prepared to do anything.

Finally, the results had come back from the lab . . . the silver dressing was working. There were signs of improvement. I should have been overjoyed at the news, but I felt unwell. I was hot and shaking, and later in the evening I was given oxygen to help with my breathing. Intravenous drips were put into my arm and blood tests were taken. I had Pneumonia. There had been an infection going around the hospital. I overheard a nurse telling a colleague there were a number of patients who had chest infections. My family was devastated, although I was too ill to care.

A week later, I recovered. The antibiotics administered were given early enough to fight the infection. Being in hospital meant the doctors were straight into action and caught the infection in the very early stages. One simple blood test told them the antibiotic I needed. Four days later, I felt great and I was hoping to go home.

I have to say, being in this particular hospital was one of the worst experiences of my life. However, it was all because of being in isolation for such a long period of time, and the thought of never going home again. For most of the time, I had convinced myself I was in a nursing home, but the hospital staff had continued to be very good and patient with me, and so were the doctors. They had, after all, saved my foot, as well as fighting a water infection which had been really hard to get rid of. I was clever enough to know that only a few years ago I would have died from at least one of my ailments. I realised this hospital was a good place to be when you're very ill, and not an institution for people who had been given up on, as I had thought. There were doctors on the wards all the time, and they came to see me on a daily basis. My family all commented on how the doctors always took time to explain to them what was happening. If you were to ask a nurse, then she would get the doctor to speak to you. It was never too much trouble. Both Geoff and Tony had said from the start they had some really good doctors at the hospital, and felt confident they could make me well again.

The man in the room next to mine had driven me mad over the last couple of months. He was also in isolation. He would shout all the time for the nurses, and it must have been as irritating for them as it had been for me. The nurses were constantly going into his room to ask him to stop shouting. One day, I snapped and shouted "Shut up for Christ sake, I'm sick of bloody hearing you." It seemed to have worked, he was quiet for a few hours, but the yelling soon started again. I would shout to tell him to shut up, and he would tell me to shut up back, and so it went on.

I was having an argument with a stranger through a wooden wall.

Sitting in my chair a few days later, still waiting to be discharged, I had seen a lot of activity going off. Margaret told me most of the wards were being shut down, but she didn't know why. I wasn't allowed to go out onto the corridor anymore, and had to stay in my room, and Teresa said there was also a nasty smell of faeces drifting around the hospital. When Geoff arrived the following morning to give me a shave, I heard him ask the nurse if they were shutting the wards down because of a virus. The nurse told him there was a bacterial infection going around the hospital, but wouldn't say what sort of infection it was. This bothered Geoff.

'If it's the superbug C.Diff, then I want my father-in-law home. He's already very nearly lost his foot through the MRSA he contracted in the last hospital. He's caught a pneumonia infection in this one, possibly from the MRSA, and if he gets this superbug, it will almost certainly kill him. I think we need to look at you letting him go home very soon.'

Geoff explained to the nurse he wasn't angry with the hospital. After all, it wasn't their fault, and they had worked hard to fight the ongoing water infection, which was probably made complicated because of the MRSA, as well as finding the correct medication for my Parkinson's. He was just frightened for my safety. We all knew my body couldn't take anything else. The nurse was very understanding.

'You'll have to see the consultant and discuss the problem with her. I can't make that decision'

'Thank you. How long will she be?'

'She has a ward round to do. You could be waiting a few hours.'

'That's OK, I'll wait.'

'You'll have to wait at the end of the corridor away from the wards.'

'That's fine. I don't mind waiting as long as I have to, just as long as I see someone. I appreciate you're all very busy, even more so now.'

Geoff told us all later how he waited until the specialist had finished her rounds, and how he was shown into her office at the end of the ward. The doctor started off by saying that she was pleased with the way I had improved since coming onto her ward, and how she hoped to be able to let me come home very soon. She also pointed out this was subject to my continued improvement. Geoff asked her what criteria she was using to base her judgement on. Was it on my hospital records or from information gathered from the reports of my Parkinson's specialist? The doctor explained she was taking into account how I had looked to her when she first saw me admitted to the ward, and the results of the investigations she and her team had carried out. Geoff agreed there had been significant improvement in my condition, and thanked her for her dedication to making me well again.

He then explained that before I was admitted to casualty in the previous hospital, I had been walking normally. In fact, I had been walking Bonny around the playing field, and joining in our trips out and about. He told her I had been travelling in the car, and even managing a holiday in France only months before. Geoff went on to describe how prior to my water infection, I had watched and enjoyed, among other programmes, Question Time and local and national news bulletins. He then asked the doctor if she felt the man she had first seen was someone who could have been competing with his daughter, to be the first to answer the questions on the Saturday night Lottery quiz show?

The specialist was surprised at this description of my previous state of health and Geoff took the opportunity to force home his point.

'I know when you first saw Patrick he was extremely ill, and his cognitive powers were seriously impaired. He found it very difficult to be coherent and often his mind seemed to be very muddled as if he was far away, so I need to ask you one question.

Would the onset of dementia, or say Alzheimer's disease, develop so intensely and in a matter of weeks?'

'No, not normally, as a rule there is a slow progression of the symptoms, Mr. Millar's condition is certainly down to Parkinson's, and the fact that he has been suffering from a very severe water infection' the Consultant confirmed.

'I agree' said Geoff 'and it's because he is out of his normal environment. He is frightened and bewildered by everything that is happening to him, and he is convinced he has been put into a home. He has this belief that people who go into a home; die.'

The specialist agreed the situation in hospital was often confusing to elderly people, and how it was their policy to get them back into their own homes as soon as possible. She explained that she was satisfied I had made significant improvements, and she was almost ready to discharge me. Geoff said quickly.

'If Patrick catches this new bug which is spreading on the ward, he may never get a chance to come home. We have everything we need at home to look after Patrick on our own. We have really good doctors, and our GP is quite happy to provide anything he may need medically.'

Geoff was informed by the Consultant that a social worker would have to visit my home before I was allowed out. They had to ensure the house was suitable for my needs. When he asked when the social worker would be able to come and view the house, she said it would be a week or so. Geoff explained to the doctor how I had been cared for at home over the years, and told her of the alterations he had made. The doctor thought that was good enough, and would inform social services I was to be considered well enough to return home.

Another problem came up. Transport wouldn't be available until the following Tuesday, my heart sank as it was only Friday, and I was worried I might not be able to go home if something else happened. I heard little bits of the conversation between Geoff and the nurses, something about a taxi that had wheelchair access. Geoff said goodbye to me, and told me he would be back later.

With all the strength I had in the world, and with the heavy dressing still on my foot, I forced myself out of the chair and limped after him. My foot hurting like hell, I shouted out to him to take me home. Geoff hadn't heard me, he was in a hurry. The nurse ran after me down the corridor, to prevent me going anywhere near the other wards. She was surprised how fast I was moving, and gently took me back to my room. My foot was very sore, I could have cried with the pain. I sank down in my chair not knowing quite what was happening. Just one hour later, Geoff arrived with my wheelchair, and it had yellow ribbons tied to it. I watched Geoff pack my bag. I took one last look around the room, and a lump came into my throat. I was on my way home. When the taxi arrived outside of the house, I could see through the car window, it was very emotional. All my family was there waiting at the door, and the garden had yellow ribbons hanging on the bushes. I was home.

The following week a social worker came to see me. She was a really nice woman, who asked about our living arrangements, and whether I had to climb the stairs to go to bed. She also asked if we needed carers to wash and dress me.

Jaysus, what an awful thought.

Geoff walked into the room at this point and told her we managed fine on our own. He also told her of the urgency there had been to get me home.

'My father-in-law has been home for just over a week. We brought him home before he caught the C Diff bug; it seems to be affecting a lot of the elderly, so it's just as well we did.'

The social worker agreed.

'Well if he's ok, then that's fine, if you need anything just let me know.'

A lot of changes had to be made. I had open bed sores on my bottom, elbows and feet, and there was still the possibility that I was carrying the MRSA bug. Geoff decided it was too much for Margaret to cope on her own, especially now. He made the final decision to care for me full time. He had already cut the days he worked down to just a couple, and he told the firms he worked for that he wouldn't be able to continue to work for them anymore, and explained he was needed at home.

I was so grateful to be home again, but from walking Bonny around the field, and being able to walk upstairs unaided, I was now quite restricted in my movements. Geoff asked the occupational therapy lady if we could have a stair lift because it was hard for him to help me walk upstairs, but she said no; her argument was simple.

'It's too dangerous for your father-in-law. We don't allow patients with illnesses such as Parkinson's disease to use stair lifts. It's for the safety of the patient.'

Geoff stated his case.

'But he will never use it on his own. He is never left by himself, what are we supposed to do?'

'I'm sorry, but that's how it is. They have to be able to operate the lift themselves. If he can't get upstairs by himself, then he will have to sleep downstairs. The only other option is a nursing home.'

Geoff was very angry, and said to Margaret he would start to look for a second hand stair lift. The following day, he went to look at some which were advertised, but they were old fashioned and tatty. We couldn't possibly afford a new one; they were over a thousand pounds. However, after a few days of searching, he managed to find a stair lift that had only been used a month before the lady went into a home. In less than a week of being refused a stair lift, I had one fitted and working. Geoff fitted it all by himself. It certainly made my life easier. I often made excuses to go upstairs for something; just for the fun of using it. When I reached the landing, I pressed a button and the chair spun round and faced me in the right direction.

I was quite capable of using the stair lift on my own. It wasn't difficult to operate.

The District Nurses came every other day to change the dressings on my sores, and I still had trouble walking due to the pressure on

130

my foot. I overheard Geoff telling the nurse how the smell of rotting flesh was bad, especially when the dressings were removed. The whole house must have smelt terrible, because candles were constantly being burned, and I knew Margaret always burnt candles to get rid of nasty smells rather than using anything out of an aerosol can. I was given blow up bags to rest my feet on and keep any pressure off the mattress, but healing was not yet in sight. Learning about pressure sores helped Geoff to understand what was needed to help the nurses with my treatment. One of the district nurses talked Geoff through how a pressure sore develops.

'Pressure ulcers can develop when a large amount of pressure is applied to an area of skin over a short period of time, or as in Patrick's case they can also occur when less pressure is applied over a longer time. The pressure disrupts the flow of blood through the skin, and the affected skin becomes starved of oxygen and nutrients, and begins to break down, leading to an ulcer forming. Patrick's heels are very vulnerable because they have so little soft tissue between the bone and the skin. This means there is very little to absorb the pressure. It's like the tissue is being squeezed between the bone and the skin, and this cuts of the blood supply, allowing the tissue to die and become ulcerated.'

'So you're saying the sore develops on the inside as well as on the outside'

'That's right; it's too late by the time you see the bruising. The damage is done.'

The nurse explained how she was going to treat my sores. She said she was going to apply a dressing of seaweed which would help to speed up the healing process. After they had both washed their hands, they propped my leg up with pillows, so that my heel was well off the mattress. The two of them put on gloves that came out of a sealed package, and spread out all the things they needed onto a large yellow sterile sheet, which was also in the pack.

'It's really important to keep everything sterile, because we are going to go deep inside the wound.' The nurse said unwrapping another green pack.

I was really glad I couldn't see it. It was bad enough having to bear the pain, and I knew I would have been sick at the sight of all that dead tissue.

'Sorry about this Patrick, we're just going to clean it all up. I know it must be painful, but we will be as quick as we can.' The nurse said to me, before turning back to Geoff. 'We use this sterile water and the swabs to gently wash the infected area, before we apply some of the seaweed compound to the smaller lint pad, and place it directly onto the wound. It will help to break up the dead tissue, so we will be able to remove it. Now all we need to do is cover Patrick's heel with this specially designed dressing, and we're done.'

Once again she apologised to me for causing me pain, and cleaned everything away before going through the exact same routine on my other heel. The nurse explained they didn't want any cross infection, and that she had swabbed both wounds to, once again, check for MRSA.

Now that both heels were finished they were going to start on my bottom.

Geoff asked how common pressure sores were, because one of my heels had a hole in it the size of his thumb.

'They're much more common in older people, or if someone has been bed bound for a long time. Two out of three of the people we see are seventy or over. This is because they are less likely to move around, and their blood and skin are much thinner. In fact, they really need checking on a regular basis to make sure sores are not developing.'

'He certainly moves around here. He hasn't had any sores at all. We're always keeping him moving,'

'I know you are. He's very well cared for.'

The district nurses continued to come for some time until Geoff suggested that he could clean and apply the dressing himself. He had been watching and helping the nurses, and it meant we did not have to wait for them to come before I could get out of bed. The leader of the nursing team agreed that Geoff could change the dressing twice a week and they would call once a week to check on my progress.

I missed being able to walk as I had done before my long stay in hospital, and I found it very hard to accept that Christmas had been and gone, and I had no memory of it. I hadn't been outside for some time, and began to feel I never would. I refused to go out in a wheelchair for all the neighbours to see. The sores on my foot made it hard to walk, the sores on my bottom made it hard to sit, and the sores on my arms and elbow made it hard to lie down. The memory foam mattress made sleeping a little better, but it didn't have the same effect as the air bed had in hospital. Moving in bed was very difficult. The sores would rub and then bleed. Fresh bedding was put on the bed daily with a pack of padding for my heels. Margaret and Geoff decided that something needed to be done, so Margaret telephoned the lady from Social Services. She asked if I could be supplied with an air bed, similar to the one that had been so comfortable during my long stay in hospital. Margaret suggested it was the least they could do, particularly as it was the treatment I had received in the first hospital ward, and my long wait in casualty, which had caused the sores and MRSA in the first place. The lady sympathised with our predicament, but informed Margaret that it was policy to only supply hospital beds and air mattress to terminally ill patients.

Once again I was refused.

Margaret sensed I was feeling down. She held my hand.

'Come on, let's use some guided imagery, I use this sort of thing in hypnosis.

Close your eyes; take a deep breath in and then breathe slowly out . . . now with each and every breath you take, you'll find yourself feeling more and more relaxed . . . that's right. . . Just let go . . . there's nothing to bother you now. Every muscle in your body is feeling more comfortable . . . from the top of your head; to the tips of your toes. This is a special time, a time for you . . . a time to relax, a time when nothing else matters. You may hear other sounds around you . . . but these sounds will only add to the feeling of relaxation, because nothing bothers you now. You are feeling so comfortable and so relaxed, your shoulders no longer feel heavy . . . and all that tension has gone.   And you feel completely relaxed.

I'm going to take you on a little journey.   Listen to the sound of my voice and let your mind just wonder where it will . . . you don't even have to listen to my voice really.   It's your sub conscious mind that I'm speaking to now. That part of your mind that knows everything about Patrick.

We were all born with the wonderful power of imagination and I want you to use your imagination now . . .

It's almost springtime. Use your power now and imagine you're outside in the garden . . . you're sitting beneath a brightly coloured parasol on a comfortable chair . . . drinking a nice cup of tea . . . the birds are singing . . . you can hear the sound of someone using a lawn mower in the distance . . . a gentle comfortable sound of spring. Bonny is rolling in the grass and you have a sense of well being . . .

Those long days you spent in the hospital are in the past now . . . just a distant memory . . . a memory that will fade away in time.   A memory you no longer need in your life.

You feel much better now . . . in body and in mind.

There's a gentle breeze brushing against your skin . . . you look up at the trees softly blowing to and fro. The garden is slowly starting to wake from its long winter sleep . . .

And as you tilt your face upwards, you can feel the morning sun penetrating throughout your body . . . healing, as the warmth of the sun runs down from the top of your head to the tips of your toes . . . you can feel the touch of Bonny, as she nudges against your knee, asking if you're walking her today.

You stand up nice and tall and slowly walk down the garden path, towards the back gate that's leads to the field, the field where you have walked with Bonny many times before.

Just a few yards . . . as you know you have to take your time now. But you can walk . . . you will walk . . . you are determined to walk.

You are gaining strength to do this every night as you sleep, and you will remember this scene in your mind, and bring this visualisation into a reality.

Very soon, I'm going to count from 1 to 5 and bring you back into the here and now. When you wake you will feel refreshed, fully alert and wide awake, and very happy.

1 . . . 2 . . . 3 . . . 4 . . . 5 and you're wide awake and fully alert.'

I had felt very relaxed after what seemed to me to be a few minutes; but turned out to be thirty minutes. Margaret's voice had been slow and very quiet. I had experienced a strange sensation, as if I was floating. I could actually feel the warmth from the sun penetrating my skin. To think I had always thought it was mumbo jumbo.

About a month later, I was sitting in the garden drinking tea. The sun was shining, although there was still a little nip in the air. Bonny was rolling in the grass, the sun was warming my body, and I suddenly remembered the hypnotherapy session. Margaret had told me to imagine this scene.

I did eventually walk again, and I took Bonny out in the field, not as far as I once had, but I brought my dream to reality. However, it was to be a year before my bedsores were to heal completely; I had to have large plasters that hurt like hell when they were being taken off. Nonetheless, with a lot of perseverance, the sores gradually reduced in size until they were only a slight discolouration, but though they had healed, it was vital that they were not subjected to sustained pressure.

Chapter Nine

Am I Dying

(2008)

Apart from the early days, when my Parkinson's medication seemed to make me sleep a lot, I never slept during the day. Not that I did much sleeping during the night either. I seemed to drift off for two or three hours, before spending time fully awake until the cycle repeated itself. There were, however, occasions when I was resigned to staying in bed all day. On these rare times, which were usually due to an infection, Margaret would put music on for me.

'You need to rest today Dad, to give the antibiotics a chance to heal your body. Shall I put some Enya music on for you?'

'Yeah, that'll be great.' I would reply, though I couldn't remember who Enya was until she started to sing. The soft sound of the singer's voice would immediately send me into a relaxed state, and I would fall into a comfortable sleep every time. When Margaret thought I had slept long enough, she would play more upbeat music or Irish music where I knew the words.

'Time to wake up Dad, you won't sleep tonight if you have too much in the day.'

Then one morning the strangest thing happened.

'Good morning Paddy. I've a nice cup of tea here for you. Wake up. Paddy . . .'

I heard Geoff leave the room and shout for Margaret to come straight away, as I wasn't responding. She rushed into my room, knelt beside me and cried frantically.

'Dad, Dad, wake up. Can you hear me?'

I could hear her, but I couldn't respond. They knew I was aware of their presence because of the tears running from my eyes. After spending a while trying to get me to come round, Margaret asked if I could move my finger to indicate a 'yes'.

'Can you hear me dad'?

I move my finger 'yes.'

'Can you open your eyes?'

I didn't reply, and at that point I realised she hadn't given me a signal to indicate a 'no'!

'Are you in pain?' I didn't reply.

'Dad, do you know who I am?'

Once again, I moved my finger and my chin quivered as more tears started to run down my face, and I could taste the salt on my lips. A slight feeling returned, and I was able to nod my head, but I still couldn't open my eyes, neither could I speak.

The ambulance arrived and I heard them mention the word 'Stroke'. However, after checking me over, they said it didn't appear to be a stroke and my pulse, blood pressure and temperature were normal. They started shouting my name and asked me to open my eyes, and I suddenly got the impression they thought I was pretending. It seemed obvious to me from the sound of their voices that they weren't sure what to do.

'What do you want us to do with him? Do you want us to admit him to hospital?'

'I'm not sure what to do' Margaret said, 'he needs to take his Parkinson's medication as soon as possible.'

Immediately the paramedics realised the problem may be associated with Parkinson's disease, but they were still undecided about what to do. Eventually, they agreed to take me to hospital just to be on the safe side, and Margaret argued which hospital I should go to.

'I don't want him going back to the local hospital, can you take him to the hospital in West Yorkshire.'

The ambulance men explained it was out of their jurisdiction, but Margaret stood her ground and said she would take me herself. I could hear the men being sympathetic with her, explaining that if something happened on the way there, she wouldn't be able to live with herself. Margaret started to cry at this point, and told the paramedics how I went into hospital with a water infection and came out in a wheelchair, three months later after recovering in a rehabilitation hospital. They listened as she told them how I had contracted bedsores, from the long stay on a casualty trolley, and how she wasn't prepared to let it happen again. The two men went outside for a discussion and eventually told Margaret they were going to take me to the hospital in West Yorkshire.

Bringing in their portable chair, they lifted me from my bed and I suddenly open and closed my eyes. I don't know why it happened, it just did. By the time they had prepared me for going into the ambulance, I was fully aware of what was happening, and was able to open my eyes properly. The paramedics decided to take me to the hospital just the same, to be certain there wasn't some underlying reason for what had happened.

When we arrived at the hospital, Margaret and Geoff thanked the paramedics for being so understanding. I was wheeled into a side ward in the casualty department, and it was only a few minutes before a doctor came and examined me. He discussed a few details with Margaret and Geoff, and decided to do some tests. When he examined me, he noticed I was still very tender from my previous bed sores. They had a different policy for elderly patients in this particular hospital. A specially designated team appeared, as if from nowhere, consisting of a doctor, two nurses and three or four auxiliaries. They checked me over from head to foot, and asked me a lot of questions about how I managed at home. Whether I could feed myself, and did I manage to go to the bathroom on my own.

When they saw the remnants of my pressure sores, the doctor turned to one of the auxiliaries and said.

'We are going to need an air mattress.'

Off went the auxiliary nurse and within five minutes she was back carrying a large blue bag. Once they had opened the bag, it wasn't long before a small electric pump was blowing up a great big blue mattress.

Before very long they had given me a bed bath, dressed me in my pyjamas and checked me over completely. Escorted by the whole team, I was taken to the ward where they handed me over to the nursing staff and I was made comfortable. Geoff had been with me all through this procedure, as he needed to help me with some of the questions which were being asked. He asked if he could stay with me and help, as he had done in the last hospital, but the nurse said that usually no one was allowed on the ward during meal times, including doctors. She went on to explain.

'The nurses make sure the patients are eating, and will help them if necessary. They also ensure the patients drink plenty of fluids by keeping a record of what drinks are consumed, and how much urine is passed.'

However, as Geoff was used to looking after my needs, and was used to my Parkinson's medication, they agreed he could stay.

I was in the hospital for a week before being allowed home. Unfortunately, no one seemed to know why I been unable to open my eyes on that morning, and assumed it was a problem associated with having Parkinson's disease. The doctors said it was probably due to the signals from my brain.

Over time, my catheter was also to cause many problems. Regrettably, the tap at the end of the leg bag was prone to catching on the hem of my trousers. It was a lever tap to make it easy to open and close, so I had to wear a special tubular bandage. The tap tucked inside of it, but the bandage kept rolling down, and the tap would pop out again. Margaret and Geoff were always checking it and usually caught it in time, before the tap opened up completely. Sadly, on one occasion the tap opened while I was in my bedroom, and the contents of the leg bag drained all over the bedroom carpet. Having MRSA in my urine meant things had to happen fast. The carpet had to be disposed of very carefully, and couldn't just be taken to the tip.

Geoff said he thought the tap was ideal for someone who was in hospital, or bed bound, but was too easy to open if someone was more mobile. Up to now we have replaced the carpet in my bedroom twice, the carpet in the lounge and two mattresses. At first our insurance company were very understanding, but it was their policy to only pay out on the first two carpets. Margaret and Geoff were annoyed at this; after all we had paid extra for accidental damage and, worse still, from now on the policy would have the accidental damage section removed. Ironically the insurance was with 'Age Concern'. Later, the design of the tap was changed to a push through version, which was much more secure and much less prone to coming open.

Whenever we went anywhere for a day out, we always had the problem of where to empty my catheter. Geoff didn't like to use public toilets because of the possibility of infection to me, or others from having MRSA in my bladder. There were no specialised places to do such things, so Geoff had to bring a bottle, find a private place and empty the contents of my urine bag into it. Of course there was nowhere to discard the bottle, so it had to be wrapped tightly in a plastic bag until it could be disposed of safely. Wherever we went, it was always a problem.

*

This was the year Margaret started to write a book that no one knew about. When she was half way through writing her book, she decided to show Geoff. He was amazed when he read it, and immediately set about enquiring about publication. It was also the year she started University. We were all surprised when she had been accepted, as she had no previous academic qualifications. She said anyone could do the therapies she had been doing, and going to University would be a dream come true. After an appointment with someone at the University, she was told she had been accepted. We were all delighted to hear the news and she started at the end of September. Margaret loved University life from the first day and suddenly there were books and papers everywhere.

She was working most of the time studying for her degree, and to make sure I wasn't spending too much time on my own, she would sit at the table and I would sit opposite her, far enough away from her, so as not to spill a drink on her books. Here, I would sit, listening to music, and reading the paper, or fiddling with anything that was nearby. One day I was fidgeting so much, trying to reach some papers she had on the table that she suggested we went into the front room, where she could sit beside me while I watched a film. Margaret helped me settle down on the sofa next to where she was going to sit, turned the volume down low, and made us both a cup of tea; placing mine in front of me on a little table within easy reach. She started on her work, typing away at the laptop which was on her knee, when all of a sudden I screamed at the top of my voice. I had spilled a full cup of tea all over my privates. I was soaked. Margaret quickly put the computer out of the way and came rushing back with a towel.

'You're wet through. We're going to have to get you out of these clothes. I hope you haven't scalded yourself, although the tea wasn't very hot, but you can't sit in those wet clothes. I have no idea what time Geoff will be back.'

'I feel wetter still now it's gone cold.'

Margaret laughed.

'Yeah, it's funny how something cold always feels wetter than something warm. I'll bring a chair in from the dining room, and try to slide you across to sit on it, while I work out how to get you changed. I can't do anything where you're sat now. I'll go and get a bath towel to cover you and keep your dignity, while you stand up and hold onto me.'

The problem with sitting on a sofa is getting up again, and I knew she had placed me there for a reason, so she could get on with her work. It was to stop me constantly trying to stand up from my chair and her fearing I would fall. It was impossible to try and stand where I was sat. The deep soft leather cushions meant I needed two people to lift me.

Margaret didn't like to ask for help from the neighbours, she knew I wouldn't want them to see me like this, so she struggled to get me off the sofa herself. Somehow, with much effort, she managed to get me onto the dining chair. My shirt and vest were also soaked from being tucked in my trousers, so she took those off first and helped me put a clean vest and shirt on.

'I'm going to have to ask you to stand now Dad. You can hold onto my shoulders while I take your trousers and boxers off. It's important we don't pull on the catheter tube, so we have to be very careful. Your shirt front will drop down when you stand, so you don't have to worry about me seeing anything.'

She took off my shoes, and I stood up from the chair, holding onto Margaret's shoulder while she unfastened my trousers. Margaret carefully slid them down my thighs avoiding pulling on the catheter tube. I sat down again while she gently pulled the trousers over my feet. The second time I stood, for my boxers to be removed, wasn't as successful; somehow I lost my balance and fell over to the side, bringing Margaret down with me. I lay half on the sofa and half on the floor. Margaret seemed to have fallen straight over the chair and onto the floor. To some, this may have been a disaster, but not in this house! Neither of us could stop laughing, and it took a while to compose ourselves. She stood up, brought the chair to its standing position and helped me sit on it again. At that very moment Geoff walked through the door with my son Patrick. Margaret told them what had happened and we laughed again.

There were many more times to come when both Margaret and I had the embarrassment of her having to undress me, or help with my toilet needs. However, we had a good system where I was covered by my shirt front or by any other means.

'Dad, we have to get on with it. We don't want outsiders coming in, do we? When these gloves are on my hands, I'm your carer for that short time, not your daughter. You have to think of it like that.'

Still, it wasn't always easy. I never thought it would come to this. Our roles had changed quite considerably over the years. She was the mother and I was the child. The only difference was, children are cute, and it's a pleasure to bathe and dress them, whereas I was an old man.

Usually, when I had a shower, Geoff kept my dignity by letting me dry myself as much as possible. One particular day, he noticed I was very sore where I pass water. By coincidence, the district nurse was due the same morning to change my catheter, and Geoff mentioned it to her. She had a really good look and agreed it was very sore and told him to put some cream on the soreness, using a cotton bud. The pain was terrible, especially at night when I couldn't sleep for the discomfort. One day I fell to the ground when walking to the kitchen, I was in agony. An appointment at the local hospital was made for me by my GP, and the doctor there confirmed I had a split in my penis. He said it was due to the long term use of the catheter, and was causing infections. Geoff listened to the doctor and wondered if this was the reason why I hadn't been responding to treatment for my water infections. He wondered if perhaps there could be two infections, and mentioned this to the Specialist.

'My father-in-law has constant water infections which never seem to clear up before another one occurs, could it mean he is having two different infections doctor?'

'Yes, it could well be, I'll write a prescription out for you for some antibiotic cream, as well as some tablets, that should help.'

But it didn't help. The pain was causing me great discomfort, so Geoff made enquiries as to what could be done about it, when, yet again I was back in the same hospital with another water infection. He explained to the doctor in desperation.

'My father-in law is having a water infection every few months. He's constantly on antibiotics and he has trouble walking because of the pain. Is there anything else that can be done? He can't carry on like this.'

The doctor looked at my notes and replied.

'He has a condition called, 'Iatrogenic hypospadias.' It is caused by an injury to the ventral male urethra, produced by the downward pressure of an indwelling urethral catheter.'

A what?

Geoff asked if anything could be done for the condition.

'There is an operation we sometimes use, involving a suprapubic catheter. It's an operation where we put the catheter straight into the bladder, rather than through the penis. Unfortunately, we can't take the risk of operating on Mr Millar. He has a heart condition, plus he is eighty one years old.'

'So you're saying you won't do it?'

'No, we can't take that risk.' The doctor replied, to which Margaret said.

'The Queen Mother had a hip replacement and she was going on one hundred.'

The doctor ignored Margaret's statement and continued with the conversation.

'We can give him a small dose of long term antibiotics which should help.'

A prescription was written and it was final, I had to live with it. There were times when I wished I wasn't living. It was painful to sit, stand and walk. The only relief I had was to lie down. Months passed and nothing improved, in fact it was much worse, but I won't go into details. I overheard Margaret and Geoff talking one day.

'He's not well, and he's really weak. We have to do something. We can't let him suffer like this.'

'I know.' Geoff agreed. 'I think he has another water infection, or perhaps it's the same one that won't respond to antibiotics. I recognise the signs and it's only just over a month since the last one.'

'Shall we take him to another hospital?' she asked 'The one where they were really good to him.'

144

'You can't just take him to a hospital' Geoff replied 'they won't take him in without it being an emergency, or seeing a doctor first.'

Geoff said the only thing we could do was to phone the doctor, but being a Sunday meant the surgery was closed, and it wasn't classed as an emergency to call out a locum, so we had to wait until Monday. However, the decision was taken out of their hands when later in the afternoon, on a visit to my grandson's house in West Yorkshire; I had a fall and badly grazed my hip. Although I was just about able to stand, they took me to the causality department at the very hospital they had been discussing earlier in the day.

When we arrived at the hospital, Geoff asked a passing man for assistance, while Margaret went to find a wheelchair. It was awful getting out of the car, my hip hurt, but it was the hypospadias that was the worst . . . it had a name now, but having a title didn't stop it from being really painful. I was at the stage where I didn't care what was going to happen to me. After a discussion at the front desk, they wheeled me into a side room. A doctor examined me and I was taken for x-rays. When I was wheeled back to the cubicle on the trolley, he said my hip was fine, but he was concerned about my chest and also wanted to do an ECG. I was kept in the side room where I was to have more blood tests taken. An hour or so later, a consultant doctor came back with the results. He pulled the curtain around the bed to deliver the findings. It always amuses me why doctors think a curtain will prevent the other patients from overhearing a conversation, especially when they insist on shouting to older patients instead of speaking to them.

'We'll have to admit you I'm afraid. You have a chest infection. There's also blood in your urine and we're still waiting for the test results to come back for that.'

Geoff didn't miss this opportunity.

'Can you just have a look at him down below? He's very sore.' Geoff explained in detail after Margaret left the room to give me some privacy. The consultant examined me making a Tut- Tut sound.

'My, my, Patrick, it does look sore. You must be very sore indeed. I'll get the urologist to take a look at this.'

I was admitted onto a ward and an air mattress was already waiting for me to make sure my bed sores, which were almost healed by now, didn't get any worse.

The urologist arrived in the evening, and after examining me, asked why I had to have a catheter fitted. Geoff explained I had an enlarged prostrate which couldn't be operated on. The doctor shook his head and said.

'I see, although it could also be a problem accelerated by Parkinson's. Some people find they cannot urinate, and others become incontinent. But, Patrick's problem is that he is getting infections externally from the catheter and internal water infections as well. He needs a suprapubic catheter insertion. It's a simple operation and only takes ten minutes. I will do it myself, but first we have to get his lungs and chest cleared up. However, as with any operations, there are risks and your father is a very poorly man. He will have to stay in hospital until we get everything cleared up before making a final decision.'

Both Margaret and Geoff agreed, and explained I had no quality of life as I was now, and I seemed to have one infection after another. Margaret told him if I was well enough to make the decision, she was sure I would agree.

I had been in hospital for a few days, but the infection was not going to go away, and the chest infection I had, turned out to be pneumonia. Late one evening I took a turn for the worse and was very ill. This time I projectile vomited a black liquid. It was like acid and burned my throat. From what I was told, I slept for three days after that episode. I had intravenous drips in my arm when I woke up, and blood was constantly being taken for tests. Oxygen was being introduced through a tube up my nostrils and I had a nebuliser mask on my face. My mouth was dry, it hurt to swallow, and I coughed on everything that was put into my mouth. A nurse was talking to my family. The nurse assumed I was sleeping but I wasn't asleep. I had my eyes closed because I couldn't open them again. I heard the nurse say.

'He's having trouble with swallowing. This often happens in the later stages of Parkinson's disease, and swallowing problems can increase the risk of aspiration, just like now. This can cause pneumonia, particularly in people with Parkinson's disease. It's very common at this stage of the Disease.'

Margaret jumped in quickly.

'He isn't in the later stages of Parkinson's disease, and he has no problem at all with his swallowing. He had a meal the day before he came into hospital and ate every bit without a problem. He always does. We know that because we are with him all the time. Dad enjoys his food and eats at the table with us. We understand he's very ill now, but he's suffered so many water infections over the last three years, his strength is draining away. He isn't in the later stage of Parkinson's . . . and he can hear, even though his eyes won't open.'

I wanted to tell them that whatever it was that had come out of my mouth had burned me. It was like hot metal. I couldn't swallow because it had hurt my throat.

Things turned from bad to worse. I was unable to swallow my medication, and as usual the red tablet spilled down my chest like red paint. Being unable to take my Parkinson's medication added to the problem of my body jerking violently. The spasms in my body were indescribable. Almost like having some sort of entity inside of me, and I had muscular spasms everywhere. I overheard a heated discussion between Geoff and the nurse about making sure I had swallowed my medication, and the fact that they were crushing my tablets. Geoff had always taken control of my medication at home since leaving his job, and read the leaflets thoroughly.

'His tablets have to be given at the same time every day to work efficiently. It's very important, and you have to be certain he swallows them. We've had this problem before; the Stalevo tablet melts very quickly on his tongue and stays there until it dribbles out of his mouth. If they are broken or crushed they don't have the same lasting effect. There will be a rapid surge of improvement, but it will not last through to the next tablet.'

Unfortunately, there was no other option. They had to crush them, and I couldn't swallow the tablets even when they put a disgusting 'thickener' in the water; something they put into every drink I had now. To make matters worse, the doctor said I had an infection in my bowel which had spread from my chest. I was riddled with infections and I had terrible trouble breathing. The next day I overheard a nurse say to someone else in the room.

'He'll have to take this thickener with all fluids now, he can't swallow, poor man. What an awful way to spend the rest of your life. He might have to have a PEG fitted in his stomach to feed him, if he survives this pneumonia that is. He's very poorly.'

Am I going to die? Is that what she's saying, and what the hell is a PEG?

I wanted to shout out loud.

I hear you. I can't open my eyes but I can hear you. I'm not brain dead. Don't talk about me as if I wasn't there.

After a few more heated discussions between the staff and Geoff over my medication, they decided he could stay and give me the tablets himself. At first, all my tablets needed to be crushed into powder and mixed into the thickened water. By being very patient with me and taking a lot more time then the nurses would have been able to spare, Geoff managed to get me to drink this strange combination. Gradually I was able to swallow a little easier, but it was still difficult for me to get the big red one down. It still needed to be crushed, but I managed to take the rest. Geoff came loaded with small pots of custard, and fed me the tablets, each one in a spoonful, until they were all gone. This did actually work by helping the tablets to slide down easily, and because I was getting my medication, the jerking and thrashing started to ease and then eventually stopped altogether.

*

I'm walking on a footpath by the side of a lake. The lake is in Stephens Green in my hometown of Dublin, Ireland. Joyce, my young wife and I are pushing our baby, Margaret, in a pushchair. It's a cold damp dismal day, but the sun shines through every now and then. Joyce's stomach is swollen because she is pregnant again. I can see Michael, my three year old brother, running in front of us, throwing stones into the water and turning around to laugh every so often. Suddenly, Joyce stops walking and holding onto my arm she cries.

'I want to go home Paddy, I want to go back to England. I can't stand it here any longer, please take me home, I miss me mam.'

I look at her pretty face, her eyes pleading with me to take her home.

'I will take you home Joyce, I promise,' I say to her 'as soon as the baby is born and I've saved enough money for the passage.'

The weather is freezing cold and her nose is red. Her eyes are glazed over from a mixture of tears and the icy wind. Michael is shouting over to us. He is telling us to watch how far he can throw a stone across the water. I say to Joyce.

'He'll miss us when we leave. He's like a brother to Margaret.'

Joyce nods sympathetically.

'I know he will Paddy, but coming here was a mistake, we're moving from one lodging house to another, just like we were in England. I want to go home.'

I look over to Michael and wave, and tell him not to go too near the edge of the water. He waves back laughing, daring to go nearer still to the edge. His foot slips and he loses his balance, stumbling head first into the lake. There's an almighty splash and he disappears. Joyce is crying out to me to hurry before he drowns. I quickly run and jump into the water after him. The water is black, all black. I'm disorientated in the dark and look up to see two people dressed in blue uniforms. They are stood on the banking, looking down on me. I don't know if they are men or women, they have no faces. Standing behind them is another figure. A tall figure, dressed in a black hooded cloak. He's laughing at me and pointing to the water. I go further down and can see Michael at the bottom of the lake holding his arms out to me. I'm swallowing water; drowning, dying. I can't breathe, I can't breathe. I feel my *lungs flooding with water and I look up for help. I'm dragged out of the water and someone places something over my nose and mouth. I'm panicking over my young brother down there in the water. Another figure takes hold of me and injects something into my arm which makes me lash out. I try hard to shout, but my mouth won't let the words out.*

I open my eyes to see two nurses, one on either side of me. I put my hand to my mouth and feel an oxygen mask.

'Are you all right Patrick?' the nurse says, 'I think you were dreaming, you were shouting out. You have some fluid on your lungs, and I'm just putting a new drip into your arm. You need to wear this nebuliser to make it easier for you to breath. Try to hold still for me now, just for a few more minutes, we're almost there.'

Geoff arrives early in the morning to give me my medication, and I long to tell him about my nightmare.

'Morning Paddy, its March the 17th. It's Saint Patrick's Day. There's some football on the television tonight and the nurse says it's all right for you to have a drop of Guinness.' He smiles. 'We'll still have to put thickener into it, but you'll still enjoy it, I'm sure.'

That evening Geoff handed me the Guinness, and it did taste all right, but I was still riddled with pain throughout my body.

Neither Margaret nor Geoff believed I was going to die, and kept talking about what we were going to do when I was home again. Geoff was there from morning until the end of visiting in the evening, helping me with my medication, my meals and trying to keep my legs supple. He came every day and Margaret, being at University, came in the evenings along with the rest of the family.

Occasionally, I did have nice dreams. Sometimes I dreamed of Joyce smiling at me. She was all in white and looked as she did when she was a young woman. There was that same mischievousness about her. The way she laughed and floated about the room.

'You're not ready for coming over here yet Paddy.' She smiles 'You're getting better now. It'll be a few years yet, but I'll be here when the time comes, waiting for you.'

She floated up towards the ceiling and was gone.

'Joyce, Joyce,' I cried.

I started to feel a little better, and it was time for physiotherapy. Two young girls came into the room and one of them was from Dublin. She had a strong Irish accent and both of them were very pleasant. They began by asking how I was feeling, and asked if I thought I could do a few exercises. Geoff explained we had been doing pushing exercises with my legs while I'd been lying in bed. He would stand at the foot of the bed, and I would try to push his hand away with my feet to straighten my legs. We had been doing this for some days now and I could feel the benefit of the exercises. He suggested I might be ready to try getting out of bed, but the two physios looked shocked.

'He has been in bed for a few weeks now, and it will be difficult for him to stand and keep his balance.'

Geoff told them about how, when I came out of the rehabilitation hospital, I had been unable to walk without a Zimmer frame and that by doing these exercises, and with sheer determination, I had managed to walk on my own again. The Irish girl said.

'I'll go and bring a walking frame and we will see how we get on.'

When they left the room, Geoff whispered to me.

'Come on Paddy, if you can manage to sit on the edge of the bed and stand up with the frame, they might let you take a few steps and then we can get out of here.'

The physios came back with a frame and adjusted it for my height. They helped me to swing my legs round so I was sitting on the edge of the bed. However, I couldn't manage to stand up from the bed. I was unsure of myself and thought I might fall. The young Irish girl said to me.

'Come on Patrick, we won't let you fall, just try to put your weight onto your feet.'

I pushed with all my might and managed to straighten my legs. Both the physios held me by the arms and I moved my left foot forward. I remembered how, in the Irish army, we had always started with; 'by the left quick march,' so when I moved forward, my right foot started to follow suit. I was walking, and everyone was praising me and telling me how well I was doing. After a few steps the physios guided me back to the bed, but instead of putting me on it, they sat me down in a big chair, saying.

'Well done Patrick, we will soon have you ready for home.'

I looked at Geoff and saw he had a big grin on his face.

Eventually, I was told I could leave the hospital and was looking forward to going home. I was on a short list for the suprapubic operation that was hopefully going to improve my life. I was dressed and sat in the chair when I heard a commotion. It was Geoff arguing with the ward sister who was holding a sheet of paper in her hand. Apparently, I was allowed to go home, but not to my home, to a rehabilitation hospital. The very rehabilitation hospital I spent nearly three months in. It had come as a shock to both Margaret and Geoff too.

'He's not going back in there,' Geoff said very firmly. 'Not that I don't think it's a good hospital, it is a very good hospital, but because he will die if he goes back there. He tried to kill himself by hiding his medication.'

Geoff explained how it wasn't the fault of the nurses and how it happened. 'He lost the will to live. We can look after him ourselves.'

'I'm sorry Mr. Foster, but you will have to agree to this and sign it before he is released from the hospital. He needs to learn to walk again, and there are doctors there if he needs one, he is still a very poorly man. It's the hospital's policy, and we have to make a decision as to where would be best for him to go.'

'He'll be even worse if he goes back there' Margaret said, 'he believed he was in a home, and because he still has MRSA, they'll put him straight into isolation again. I know he's been in a single room here, but it was only a few weeks, being in isolation almost drove him mad. He can't go back in there.'

'I do understand what you are saying, but I can't see how you will be able to manage?' the ward sister argued with Geoff.

'We managed before. When he came out of rehabilitation last time, he could hardly walk; in fact he was worse than he is now. Besides, there must be a mobile physiotherapist who could come to the house and help with his walking. We have excellent doctors who will be more than happy to look after his medical needs.'

'Have you got an air bed and hoist for him?' The sister asked.

'No,' Geoff replied 'we were told they only issue a hospital bed and an air mattress to people who are terminally ill. We have a memory foam mattress, but it has never been suggested that we need a hoist.'

'Leave it with me.' The ward sister said, 'I will write to your local hospital and make arrangements for the equipment to be delivered to your home. In the meantime we will show you how to move Patrick with a hoist, should the need arise.'

She was as good as her word, and wrote a letter insisting we were provided with the equipment we needed, and for a physiotherapist to come and help me to walk properly. I didn't realise ward sisters held so much influence, but it seems if they are not happy with an outcome, they can refuse to discharge a patient.

Oh, it was so grand to be in my own home, the warmth, nice meals and the sheer comfort of my own bed. The local hospital was looking into me having an air bed to prevent bed sores, one which had different positions. It would take a few weeks, but for now I was pleased to sink into the comfort of the bed I had. While I was in hospital, Margaret and Geoff had decorated my bedroom, and replaced the carpet, bedcovers and curtains with new ones.

I was never to see the room.

My bed was brought down into the front room for a couple of weeks, while they made Margaret's therapy room into a bedroom for me. I would never use the stair lift anymore to go up upstairs, or sleep in my old room. It had been proving difficult for Geoff to help me off the stair lift at the top of the stairs, even before I was admitted to hospital. They had decided it was for the best I slept downstairs now. Unfortunately, Margaret lost her therapy room, but she insisted she had enough on with being at University and writing a book. I couldn't walk properly anymore. I had trouble standing, but both Margaret and Geoff believed that I would eventually walk again.

'You'll be walking up and down the garden path again this summer, you conquered it last time, and summer is just around the corner so we have a lot to look forward to, "the show's not over until the fat lady sings"' Geoff laughed, to which Margaret replied.

'Yeah and she's anorexic at the moment.'

The new bed arrived, and Margaret's therapy room was converted into a bedroom. Both Margaret and Geoff had struggled to make my life happy and were very positive in their outlook. Everything we had come across together was sorted out, one way or another, to make my life easier. I had everything I needed to make my life happy, a television in my room, music and my own bathroom. The new bed could be raised and lowered; it also sat me up, drew my knees up to give support, and had rails on the side to prevent me from falling out. The room was bright and colourful and I always had fresh clean bedding.

At first I used to sit with both of them in the front room watching television, but when it was time for bed, Geoff was beginning to have difficulty getting me out of the chair. It was decided I would go to bed after our evening meal, before I grew too tired, which was usually about 8.00 pm by the time we finished. I wasn't happy. I felt pushed out, but soon realised they were right. The later in the evening it was before I went to bed; the more difficult it was for them to get me settled. Besides which, they needed a bit of time on their own and made sure they popped in and out all night to see me.

154

Morning arrives once more, and my routine begins with the tablets. Geoff puts them on my tongue, one tablet at a time to make sure I swallow them. As usual, he places the first tablet in my mouth.

'Drink this water Paddy before the tablet melts.'

My hands are too jerky to hold a tablet myself, by the time it gets near to my mouth I lose it. He carefully puts one tablet after the other onto my tongue. Each time he repeats himself.

'Drink the water Paddy before the tablet melts and sticks to your tongue.'

Just like before, if we're not quick enough, the big red one melts leaving a stain that runs down the side of my mouth. Sometimes it gets fast between my teeth and my lips, causing it to slowly dribble down onto my chin and my clothes. I'm completely helpless in the mornings. My muscles won't work. I want to move my arms, but they are too heavy until my medication begins to work. I have trouble holding onto a cup, and I'm given a cup with a lid that has a spout, which I'm not happy about, as it reminds me of a baby cup.

'I know it looks like a baby cup Paddy, but it's just for when you're in bed. We don't want you spilling hot tea down yourself.' Geoff tells me, sensing my disapproval. 'When you have had your shower, I'll make you a cuppa in a proper cup, and you will have a table to rest it on.'

Nodding, as he leaves the room, I deliberately turn the cup the wrong way round, and try to drink from the little hole instead of the spout, accidently spilling tea down my pyjama top and all over the bedding. Margaret appears and sees the mess.

'Oops, I'll get you a towel to put under your chin and make you another cup of tea.'

Soon, she walks back into the room holding a fresh cup of tea in the baby cup. I feel guilty now. I know they give me the cup for my own protection. Margaret raises me further up with a touch of a button, and I'm sat more straight.

Geoff gently helps me out of bed to take me for a shower, and when I'm dressed I'm wheeled to the table for my breakfast. I haven't spoken at all this morning. My voice is having one of its low volume days. I nod when I'm asked if I would like two Weetabix and scrambled eggs for breakfast. Outside, we can hear the new buildings being built at the back of the house where the schools were. I stir my Weetabix around the dish mixing them with milk, and making mulch, as my mind wonders away to my working life on the building sites.

I think of my mates who came over from Ireland with me, and the excitement and anticipation we felt at the first time we set foot in England. We had originally come over to England to work down the coal mines after seeing a poster that was offering work in Yorkshire. The job came with full training and accommodation and as there was very little work in Dublin, it seemed a good idea. We were sent to a place called Askern, near Doncaster in Yorkshire, for our training at the colliery. It was a lovely place to live, with a nice view overlooking a large Victorian lake. A far cry from the poor tenement blocks of Dublin city.

I was happy all right, working down the mines. I remember the first day clearly. We were taken into a room and everything was explained to us. We were shown how to put our gear on, and how to use the lamps that were attached to the tin hats we wore. Quite a lot of the men had come from mining backgrounds, and were used to hearing tales of life down the mines. To the rest of us, it was a new experience altogether. I have to admit . . . and I'm sure I wasn't the only one there, I did wonder what I was letting myself in for. We were all crammed together in the cage at the top of the pit shaft, and the older men there were smiling at us as we were lowered into what seemed like a bottomless pit. The speed of the descent was such; I thought the cage would never be able to slow down in time to stop. Suddenly, within what seemed like a few seconds, we were a thousand feet below the surface. The first thing which surprised me was the walls were painted white and there was plenty of light . . . until we went further in and saw the coal face. It was blacker than black itself. We were taken to an old seam which wasn't being worked, but was used for teaching purposes. One of the trainers spoke to us about our head lamps and asked us all to switch them off. Oh Jaysus, the darkness was hard to describe. Was this how it was to be blind? We had to learn about the dangers of walking where coal filled trucks were hurtling down, and after walking a few miles further into the mine, it was hard to straighten up, which meant we had to work on our knees.

The winter months were the worst, it was dark going to work, dark in the mine and dark when you came out of the mine. But this was what I came over to England to do and I had a wage at the end of the week. The dialect took some getting used to. I was hearing words I had never heard of before. I might as well have been in a foreign land, hearing the broad Yorkshire accent. On the first day of working, we had a break for lunch and one of the men asked if I had brought some snap. Snap? I asked. What the hell was snap? I soon learned that snap was your sandwiches, which were kept in a tin box which snapped tight shut to stop the rats from eating your food.

Unfortunately, after a while they relocated us to Barnsley, and a lot of my mates went back home to Ireland. None of us liked Barnsley after living in Askern, and to make matters worse, we were housed in Bevin huts, unlike the boarding house where we had been used to living. However, this was where I was to meet the most beautiful girl I had ever seen . . . Joyce. She worked in the canteen, and when our eyes met for the first time, I knew she was the girl I wanted to marry.

After many years of working down the mines we heard there was plenty of work on the building sites, and, along with most of my Irish mates, I moved to working outside. We worked on just about all the buildings that were going up in Barnsley at the time, moving from one job to another when they were finished. Good days they were. I was a hod carrier. I could run up those ladders with a pile of bricks on my shoulder, keeping the bricklayers supplied with bricks as they built the walls. The muscles in my arms led to my nickname 'Popeye'.

Work was easy to find in those days, but the wages were very poor. In the summer months, we worked until the sun went down, to make as much money as we could. On the other hand, the winter months were hard as we had to finish as soon as it grew dark, which on some days could be as early as 3.00 pm when the fog, or smog, I should say, set in. I remember the smog in those dark days. You couldn't see anything in front of you on those nights, and had to 'feel' your way home, often hearing people before you could see them. Bronchitis was rife, as the soot and smoke settled on your chest. You could hear the sound of coughing at a great distance, yet, there was always that eerie silence in the smog.

When it snowed, which in the 1950s was often thick heavy snow, we were all out of work until we were called for again. During the winter months we really struggled with money, or should I say, the lack of it. Along with the other people who were out of work in the winter, I would have to go on 'National Assistance' and they used to give us jobs to do such as clearing the snow from old people's paths. Most of the families on our road were miners and had free coal. When the snow settled on the roof of their houses, it melted pretty quickly because their houses were warm, whereas our house and a few of the neighbour's houses, that weren't miners, were always cold so the snow on the roof soon turned to ice. We were always short of coal, but we survived. When it grew dark, I would go down to the railway embankment with an old coach built pram, to where the coal had fallen off the wagons. If we couldn't find coal at the side of the tracks we would pinch coal from the train wagons themselves. I used to climb up the embankment and get the coal piece by piece, throw it down to the ground and then put it in the pram. There were usually other people doing the same thing, and once I picked up a great big piece of slag and threw it away. Because it was pitch black on the railway sidings, it hit me auld mate John on the head and knocked him down to the ground. John shouted out in the stillness.

'Jaysus Christ Paddy, are yis trying to kill me er what? Yis just hit me right on the bloody head.'

All of a sudden people were shushing him to keep quiet; after all, we were stealing the coal. If anyone had heard us, we would have seen the light from their torches coming our way. There were many times we had to run for it, though we knew a lot of the security men turned a blind eye; they had families themselves after all. In those days there weren't the Government benefits that the unemployed have today. It was all about survival. I had five kids to keep warm. We also needed fuel for hot water and the cooking range.

We went out looking for work early in the morning once a job had finished, dressed in our work gear, ready to start work immediately. Sometimes, we would jump on a truck, known as a 'Paddy Wagon,' due to the large input of Irish labourers, with hopes of being 'set on' there and then. Many gaffers on building sites did indeed hire men this way. In fact, on one particular morning we called onto a building site, meself and me auld mate John Keenan. We were dressed in our gear ready to work, and it was still only 7.30 in the morning and bitterly cold. The gaffer, a big overweight man saw us walking towards him, and before we even asked him for a job he shouted over to us.

'I'm full up'.

To which John replied,

'Well Jaysus, aren't you the lucky wun. Paddy and me auld self have had no breakfast yet, God bless yis.'

I had met John when we were on the cattle boat that brought us to England. He told me he was from Tipperary, and explained how he pinched an old grey mare to ride all the way to Dublin, looking for work. John didn't have a penny in his pocket at the time, and apart from a couple of loaves of bread, he hadn't eaten, up to reaching Dublin.

'Jaysus Paddy', John told me, 'I could have walked all de bloody way dere, fer de length of time de bloody horse travelled, en me poor auld arse hurt without a saddle. I could neither walk nor stand when I reached Dublin. I sold the auld horse for a few bob to get meself a cuppa tea and slice o bread and a glass o stout.'

I smile to myself as I remember John; I have many happy memories of working on the building sites. And though I was a hod carrier, I often laid bricks and remember mixing the gobo, making

159

sure it was just the right consistency. Bricks are placed side by side, end to end, and the joints are spaced so each joint is halfway along the brick below. Always making sure the mortar is spread evenly, I think to myself there is great art in the method of laying bricks, and I had taken great pride in my job . . .

'Dad what are you doing?'

My thoughts were broken as Margaret walked into the dining room and made me jump out of me bloody skin.

'You've plastered your Weetabix all over the table. It's everywhere. Look! It's all down your front as well. I'll get a cloth and clean it up.'

I came back down to earth with a bump. My mind had wondered off again to another time and another place. Margaret laughed, and I started to laugh as well when I realised what I had just done.

'Don't worry about it, it'll clean up. It's probably because you've just had a cocktail of pills that are messing up your brain. It'll settle down in a while. That's quite a lot of tablets to take in one go. God knows what they do to a person's mind.' She laughs and starts to clear the 'mortar' away.

My facial muscles have decided to work again. The pills must be working.

I have finished my breakfast and Margaret has passed me the morning's paper to read. They are amazed I can still read without reading glasses, although I do have some somewhere. My eyesight has always been good and so has my hearing. Most days my speech is quiet, but then I have always spoken softly, they say Irish people do. If I try, I can easily make myself understood, it's only on the days when my voice decides it's not going to work I have difficulty. On the good days, I find my voice and read out some of the articles and reports which are written in the paper. Some of the articles spark off discussions that really help to keep my mind active and exercise my vocal cords. Others, particularly when I'm just reading to myself, send my mind drifting off into a kind of daydream, and I find I can be deeply engrossed in whatever subject is being reported on. It can be hard to distinguish sometimes what is actually an experience and what is not.

Margaret suddenly snapped me out of my day dreaming once more.

'You're staring out into space again. I wonder what you're thinking about. I would pay much more than a penny for *your* thoughts. Come on, let's get you into the conservatory for some daylight and Vitamin D.'

Margaret brings me an orange on a small plate, with a tissue to wipe my mouth and fingers afterwards. She always insists I peel my own oranges, even though it takes a while to do.

'You need to stay as independent as you can Dad.'

I eat the orange, clean my fingers, and settle down in my chair. I look out of the conservatory window and relax, watching the birds dig out worms from the grass, and think to myself.

'How is it possible for a vitamin to get into my body through my skin, and when will I know when it's happening?'

*

The day for my suprapubic catheter operation arrived and they drove me to hospital. I never spoke a word. I was frightened of going into hospital with the possibility of being moved to a nursing home. We reached the ward, and the nurse asked Geoff if he could put my pyjamas on and put me into bed. The nurses were very friendly, but I wasn't. I sulked and refused to help Geoff take my jacket off. I had no intention of climbing into bed, or giving any assistance to Geoff. I pushed him to the limit. He had never lost his patience with me, but he did that day.

'Paddy, you're only in overnight, you're coming home in the morning. What's the matter with you? You have a right sulky look on your face and you're rude to the staff. You've also upset Margaret through your stubbornness.'

It was true, the staff had asked what I would like to eat and I didn't reply. I also had Margaret in tears. I was being selfish, I

161

know that now. The nurse suggested Geoff and Margaret leave for half an hour, while they assessed me. By the time they had come back I had been examined and given my last meal, before I was to be 'Nil by Mouth'. I had eaten fish and mashed potatoes. I ate the whole lot, including a pudding, but I was still acting like a child. I sulked when the bell rang to say visiting was over. I was almost ready to cry. I wasn't frightened of the operation itself, but the fear of not being able to go home.

The next day the operation was a complete success and hardly hurt at all. My water infections were to come to an end, apart from one or two over the years and they were so easily cleared up after a course of tablets.

Life was good again.

Chapter Ten

Ireland

(2009)

'How do you feel about going to Ireland this year Dad? Beach holidays are out of the question with the wheelchair. Anyway, sitting on a beach all day is boring. I was thinking if we went to Ireland then we could go somewhere different this time, instead of staying in Dublin. Perhaps we could go more inland and hire a cottage in the country, but still be near enough to visit Dublin and see Michael and Dina again.'

'That sounds lovely.' I replied, at the thought of seeing Michael and Dina and all the family.

'Yeah,' Margaret said, still looking at the pictures on the computer. 'I think it will be a great holiday. I'll have a word with Geoff when he gets home and see what he thinks about it.'

'We had a good holiday travelling around Ireland with yer mam, I remember that holiday.' I declared with enthusiasm.

Margaret said we wouldn't be touring as we did before, but we could still do some sightseeing. When Geoff arrived home she mentioned the holiday to him, but unfortunately, he wasn't keen on the idea.

'We would be better staying somewhere nearer to home in case we need a doctor for your dad. Look what happened in France. If he's ill again, we need to be able to get him back home. Why don't we go to Cornwall or somewhere like that, at least we'll be in our own country.'

'I know it's a long way, but at least Dad can have a rest on the ferry and he would enjoy being on the Irish Sea again.'

The debate went on for over a week. Geoff said it wasn't just the travelling but the expense of it all, being in Euro's. He stressed how expensive it was going to be, as there would be six of us now Margaret had decided it would be nice to take Nicholas, Antony and Ryan again.

'We have the price of the ferry as well as travelling expenses before we even start the holiday. Why don't we go to Cornwall? There are some really nice places that have disabled cottages.'

That word again, disabled.

I thought a decision would never be reached as brochures lay on the table. Finally Geoff gave in and agreed to go to Ireland. Particularly as Margaret wanted to do some research for the book she was writing. There were quite a few places she wanted to visit which were relevant to the book, including the Michael Collins museum in Dublin.

Since I had trouble getting in and out of cars now, a new one was ordered for me. It was a disability car. I didn't like the sound of the word; 'disability,' and disliked the fact that I was now classed as disabled. Disabled, I thought about it for a while and decided it would be good to change the word to something else. What to? What sort of name could you give someone who couldn't walk very well? My thoughts were broken when Geoff said the car would be arriving the day after. He was very enthusiastic as usual.

'You'll love this car Paddy' Geoff said looking at the brochures. 'The wheelchair wheels straight into the car. You'll be like the Pope in his pope mobile. You'll be able to see out of all the windows. It's called a wheelchair access vehicle.'

That sounds much better than a disabled car.

I nod to Geoff and say something, but it wasn't recognisable. My speech is very quiet and cannot be heard. It's almost as if my voice has lost its power, and the volume button has been turned down. Margaret and Geoff often pretend to understand me. I know that. They don't like to hurt my feelings. It is strange because a lot of the time they guess right. They often know what I had said when other people can't understand me. There are days I can speak clearly enough for everyone to know what I was saying, and there are also times when they can't shut me up; especially when we are having our evening meal. I love to talk of old Ireland and my life as a child. Let's face it; I can't remember about yesterday or the day before, still, I was very excited by the prospect of seeing my brother and his family again, and being in Dublin. The only downside was being 'disabled' and the mere thoughts of being pushed in a wheelchair filled me with dread. I was glad my dear old Ma wouldn't see me like this.

A few days before we were to go to Ireland, we were eating our evening meal and it was one of those rare times when I was very talkative. It must have been the excitement of it all. The very thought of Ireland brought back memories from years ago. Margaret and Geoff were amazed how I could still remember the orders given in Gaelic, that I learned during my time in the Irish army. I spoke of my first job as a delivery boy, or messenger boy as we were called then. One job was delivering fish in a basket which was fastened on the front of my bike. If the wind was blowing towards me, the smell of fish lingered in my nose for hours after I had delivered the goods. On the other hand, being a messenger for a bakery was different. The smell of fresh baked bread made me ravenous. I had Margaret and Geoff gasping as I told them how I nearly lost my leg, or worse still, my life, when I was a young boy. We used to jump on and off the horse drawn wagons to get a free ride, and I somehow managed to get my leg caught in the wheel. Luckily for me, a woman saw what was happening and yelled to the driver, who managed to stop just in time. I was given a clip round the head from the drayman and hobbled home to get another clip from my mother. Margaret smiled and said.

'I think you kid us half the time Paddy Millar, you've talked nonstop for a good twenty minutes. It must be all this talk of going back to Ireland that's bringing up old memories.'

The table was cleared and Margaret and Geoff went into the other room while I sat drinking my cup of tea. I overheard them discussing what the best time would be to set off to Holyhead for the boat. The telephone rang and I heard Geoff speaking to

Michael, my brother, in Dublin. I was so excited at the thought of going "home again". I'd never believed it possible that I would get to visit there again, even though I had thought about it many times over the years. I was longing to stand up and join them in the other room, and decided I would set off. I placed my hands on the table and managed to slide the chair backwards. The chair fell over onto its side and I went with it. Margaret and Geoff came rushing in to see what the noise was, to find me lying on the tiled kitchen floor in what you could call a funny position. They had learned quite a lot over the years, not only about Parkinson's disease, but also about First Aid. I had to stay in the same position until they checked me over for broken bones, even though I was in a weird position.

Although I told them I felt all right and had no pain, they decided to call for an ambulance, as I had fallen onto a hard surface. Suddenly the excitement was over. We all knew there was a chance of me being kept in hospital. Not to mention the holiday having to be called off. The ambulance arrived and the paramedics checked me over, asking Margaret and Geoff if they wanted them to take me to casualty, even though they were convinced I had no injuries. I think we startled them when we all said 'No' at the same time. Soon we were all getting off to bed, ready for an early start in the morning. I was not as tired as I normally was and as I lay there my mind seemed to drift off, back to past visits to Ireland. I was not really dreaming, it was more like it had been at the dinner table, I was remembering clearly, and my thoughts drifted to past holidays.

The last time we were over in Dublin was in 1993 when Joyce was alive. We'd toured all around the coast of Ireland with Margaret and Geoff, in a motor home. Unfortunately, we were to soon realise that motor homes were not ideal for the country roads of Ireland. We had so many punctures because of the uneven road surfaces and pot holes, as we travelled all the way down the western side of Ireland. I'd never been to the west coast of Ireland. In fact, I had never been anywhere in Ireland, before coming over to England, apart from being in Killarney when I was in the Army.

The holiday was the best Joyce and I ever had, and I was astonished by Ireland's beauty. Connemara has long been regarded as the real emerald of Ireland and Margaret loved the place. Some say keeping a Connemara stone close to your heart will bring you the luck of the Irish, so Margaret nipped out of the motor home to get a stone for each of us while Geoff stopped to look at the map. He didn't notice she had jumped out, and set off driving again. Joyce was hysterical with laughter, as she waved through the back window to Margaret while she chased after us. We travelled across to Limerick and down the coast staying where they made the film 'The Quiet Man' and in Dingle, where they made 'Ryan's Daughter.' Travelling over the Kerry Mountains was so overwhelming that Joyce almost cried at the scenery spread below us. When we arrived at Blarney castle, Margaret and Geoff climbed up the hundreds of spiral stone steps to kiss the Blarney stone, and Joyce said Margaret must have swallowed the Stone because she couldn't stop talking.

We drove all around the rest of the coastal roads making our way back to Dublin, stopping overnight at different places. My mother was at Michael's house when we arrived, and was so pleased to see us. My nephew, Alan, was getting married later that day and we had all been invited to the wedding. We had a great time. This was to be the last time I saw me mother before she died. I couldn't even attend her funeral. I was recovering from a heart bypass. Thinking of the holiday to Ireland I was about to go on, I tried to picture in my mind being pushed up O'Connell Street in a wheelchair. I very much doubted the wind on my face would be as thrilling as it had been riding a bike in my youth.

A cottage had been booked by the Killarney Lakes, with a jetty almost outside of the gate overlooking the Shannon River. Margaret and the three boys ran straight down to the water's edge as soon as the car had stopped, leaving Geoff to wheel me out of the Pope Mobile. It was a beautiful sight and I longed to run down with them. My downstairs bedroom was en-suite and had two single beds, but it had the smallest bathroom I had ever seen. It was going to be almost impossible for Geoff to help me shower after being used to so much room at home. When everything was taken inside from the car, we went into Athlone town centre to buy the food we needed, and I tried to tell them that this was where my army barracks used to be, but getting the words out was hard work, and I never did get to tell them.

I was very tired that evening. We had been travelling since early morning, and I fell asleep as soon as my head hit the pillow. During the night I woke up and didn't recognise the room. I had no idea where I was, and no memory of the last couple of days. I was in a strange room with an empty bed at the side of me. Was I in a hospital, or a nursing home, or a morgue? Was I in the rehabilitation hospital again, where I had spent three months? Silent tears ran down my face. Where was I? Where were Margaret and Geoff? I couldn't find my voice to shout. I cried on and off all night, frightened of the silence. It was so unearthly quiet. I couldn't hear the odd traffic noises that I could hear at home. There were no dogs barking in the distance or sounds coming from anywhere. It was eerily silent. I tried to think. It couldn't possibly be a hospital or a nursing home, surly there would be some sounds. The hours dragged by, and I wondered why there would be an empty bed at the side of me. Whose was it? Suddenly I heard someone moving in the next room. I tensed my muscles in anticipation as the bedroom door swung open. I was so relieved to see Geoff that I broke down crying, real sobs they were. He was very sympathetic.

'Come on Paddy, you're all right now. We're on holiday in Ireland. You were very tired last night with all the travelling. It's all been a bit much for you. Let's have a nice cup of tea before everyone gets up.'

He sounded cheerful, but I still couldn't remember the journey or the day before. My mind was a complete blank. What travelling? Geoff left the room to make a cup of tea, but carried on talking to me to reassure me he was still there.

'Margaret will be down soon, and we'll have some breakfast and go over to see Michael and Dina in Dublin. We'll sort something out for you tonight in case you wake up again.'

Margaret was very upset when Geoff told her what had happened and started to cry. She said from now on, whenever we go on

168

holiday they would make sure the place had a double bed with a single bed in the same room.

We went to Michael's house in Dublin, but I must have slept the whole time while we were there. I was so tired and can't remember anything of the visit. It seems my nephews and nieces, Michael's grown up children, Jacqueline, Stephanie and Alan, all came to see me, but I'd missed them. Margaret told me something funny though a few days later. Michael's young grandson, who was there at the time, was puzzled seeing me in a wheelchair. When he went home he asked his father who the man in the wheelbarrow was. Even passing through the streets of Dublin had no pleasure for me. I couldn't rid myself of the night I had spent wondering where I was, and had lost all interest in the holiday. I prayed to God nothing would happen like that again.

Margaret and Geoff had packed the baby alarm that we use at home.

'The baby alarms set up now, so we will be able to hear you if you call out. Just like we do at home, and I've bought a bell for you to ring. I'll put it on the bedside cabinet, where you can reach it. Seeing the bell might trigger a memory, and you will know where you are and why it's there.'

'But what if you don't hear it?'

'We will, the other half of the baby alarm is next to our bed, and I will be listening out for it.'

Fortunately, that was the only night I woke up wondering where I was, and the rest of the holiday was really good. We toured other areas and sang along to the Irish songs being played in the car. Nicholas made us laugh hysterically with his new found Irish accent. He was spot on with it. Anyone would have believed he was born there.

169

Dublin had changed so much; there were cars everywhere you looked, and thousands of people swarmed around the streets as they flocked from shopping centre to shopping centre.

Jaysus, the place had changed.

When we had left the ferry on arriving in Dublin, we had driven through the City and I was surprised to see apartments with so many windows, they looked like glass houses. I hardly recognised the old Dublin town of my youth. When we went to visit the street I was brought up in, there was only one of the original tenement houses left. The old houses have gone now; replaced by new ones.

A song came up on the CD which was playing in the car. For me, it summed everything up.

Raised on songs and stories; heroes of renown.
Are the passing tales and glories; that once was Dublin Town,
The hallowed halls and houses; the haunting children's rhymes.
That once was Dublin city in the rare old times.

Ring a ring a Rosie, as the light declines,
I remember Dublin city in the rare old times.

Fare thee well sweet Anna Liffey,
I can no longer stay,
And watch the new glass cages, that spring up along the Quay.
My mind's too full of memories, too old to hear new chimes,
I'm part of what was Dublin, in the rare old times.

Those Irish songs we played travelling around Dublin, Killarney, Galway Bay, Ross Common, and even Athenry, woke up memories of places we had been to when touring Ireland with Joyce. Of course we didn't travel as far as the South West Coast this time. The boys soon learned the lyrics and I joined in with them in my own little voice, as I sat in the back of 'The Pope Mobile.' As Geoff had said, I was high up now with plenty of windows to see out of.

170

Something that amazed us all, was the respect shown to me while I was being pushed in the wheelchair. Wherever we went, people actually looked at me and spoke, instead of avoiding eye to eye contact, often standing aside to give me more space. People acknowledged me as I passed, and the traffic would come to a halt when drivers saw us stood by the kerb, allowing us to cross the busy streets. We never had a problem finding a disabled parking space, even in the heart of Dublin City.

On our last day of the holiday, we arranged to meet Michael again, and I was feeling much better than I'd been earlier in the week when I had last seen him. I was grateful I was able to have a conversation with him over a cup of tea, which was great. I wouldn't have liked his last memory of me to be of me sat in a wheelchair, all spaced out. We had met in the Michael Collins museum which used to be part of the Irish army barracks. The courtyard looked exactly how it used to look and, Jaysus, how it brought back memories of my time in the army. Memories of years ago when I was doing my square bashing, of when we had marched through Dublin and Phoenix Park in our uniforms, how very proud I had felt to be in the Irish army; even if it had only been for a short time. In the Michael Collins museum itself, there were glass cases, and display cabinets, but once again everything was too high for me to see anything. I didn't mind too much this time, because I was glad to be with my brother again, and didn't want the visit to end.

All too soon, it was time to leave and make our way to the ferry to catch the boat back to England. Trying to put a brave face on, both Michael and I made our farewells. We were not just going through the motions of parting company, we were actually saying goodbye. I think both of us knew that this was likely to be the last time we would see each other.

It was a good holiday, but I was dreading the long journey home. Funnily enough, it didn't seem to take too long. I was fully awake on the ferry. We found some nice comfortable seating near the window, and I was able to enjoy the sea journey, and of course a glass of Guinness. I could hardly believe the journey took only a few hours. A far cry from the gruelling ten hours it used to take to

171

cross over the Irish Sea when Joyce and I were young. We arrived home just before midnight and Geoff put me straight to bed. Heaven! It was so good to be back in my own bed, in my own home. We had just managed to catch the fish shop before it closed, and I sat watching television to unwind while I ate my fish and chips, along with a cold glass of lager. One glass of lager was all that I cared for now. I could visualise Joyce smiling down on me.

'It's about bloody time Paddy Millar.'

Chapter Eleven

Keep the light upon your chest

(2010)

There are days when sometimes my mind tells me I can walk, but my body decides I can't. Fortunately, through boxing in my youth, and being a hod carrier on the building sites, my arms are still strong. I'm often able to hitch myself to a standing position and sometimes I try to make my body do as it's told. One day, while sitting in my big chair looking around the room, I started to think. If I could stand and hold my balance long enough I should be able to reach the sofa. After about three attempts, I finally managed to stand up and find the courage to let go of the arms of the chair. I made it to the sofa, falling on it, rather than sitting down on it. That was good. I had made it. Then I tried to move to the chair opposite; but it's harder to stand with only the one arm at the end of the sofa to hold onto. . . I didn't make it. I fell to the floor and the dog started to run around me barking, as she always does when I fall. Margaret recognised the bark, and knew it was a warning bark, which, strange as it may seem, is different to the barking she does for other things. If Geoff is out and Margaret can't lift me on her own, she puts a pillow under my head and tries to prop me up, makes a cup of tea for us both and sits beside me until Geoff comes home. Bonny lays her head on my legs and looks at me with soulful eyes.

On another occasion I managed to walk from the front room to the conservatory. Moving from the chair to the sofa, I was able to reach the open kitchen door. Holding on to the work surface, I took a breather and weighed up the distance to the fridge, and the door of the conservatory. With one almighty rush I passed the fridge, reached the doorway to the conservatory and passing through it, I flopped down into my chair. I heard Margaret shouting my name in panic about ten minutes later, but my voice wouldn't reach her to say where I was. The front door opened and then closed, and after few minutes, I heard her run into my bedroom, obviously panic stricken as to where I could be. Eventually, she came into the conservatory.

'My God Dad, how did you get here? I've been outside looking for you. You scared me to death.'

'Did you think I'd been kidnapped?' I laughed.

'It's not funny. I only went upstairs to change the beds. It's impossible to leave you for five minutes. I have to go back again. Do Not Move.'

There are times when I have problems falling, particularly when I try to stand unaided. Usually when I fall, it's my arms and elbows that get carpet grazes on them. My wounds need to be cleaned and dressed with little strips, which act as stitches, because my skin is so thin now it literally peels backwards. We have everything needed for first aid, and Geoff gently rolls the skin back into place before dressing it. The fact that I fall is accepted now, and Margaret laughs, telling me I'm good at falling because I always land on my butt, without my head hitting the floor. Perhaps it's because I just go down in a relaxed fashion; sliding gently to the ground, rather than violently tripping and falling uncontrollably forwards, or backwards. I try not to let falling deter me from trying to walk, and most of the time I manage quite well with my walking aids, but I do understand why Margaret and Geoff take so many precautions; especially when I'm outside in the garden.

*

It has now been quite a few months since the operation to have a suprapubic catheter fitted took place, and the transformation has been unbelievable. Apart from a couple of urine infections immediately after the operation, I have been completely clear of them, and now the district nurses only come every twelve weeks to change it. I was gradually beginning to feel much more like my old self, and wanted to join in with everything again.

One afternoon Margaret and I were sitting in the conservatory, and I was relaxing in an easy chair while she was painting her nails. When she had finished, she screwed the lid onto the small bottle and left the room. The nail varnish was hard to reach, but I managed to scrape it towards me with a newspaper, something I had learned to do a long time ago when something was out of my reach. I only wanted to look at the label on the bottle out of curiosity. Geoff came into the room a few minutes later.

'Oh Paddy, what have you done?'

What was he talking about, I hadn't done anything. I never left my chair.

'You've got nail varnish all over your hands, head and face. Not to mention all over the chair arms. I'd better get a cloth before it goes in your eyes.'

I didn't have a clue how I managed to get the nail varnish on my face. I must have rubbed it on without realising. Just as well I didn't rub my eyes as I usually do. Margaret sat with me holding my hands still making sure I didn't wipe my eyes, while Geoff went up to the chemist to get some non irritating acetone free nail varnish remover. The nail varnish took a long time to remove from my skin, and scrub as much as they could; it wasn't coming off the chair arms. Geoff couldn't believe how much of the stuff could come out of such a small bottle. They decided the chair would have to be thrown away, and Geoff sawed it into bits and took it to the rubbish tip.

I couldn't blame the dog this time, she wasn't in the room.

I couldn't blame the dog either when, sat in my reclining chair, I gently dipped the chair's remote control into a cup of tea. The cup was sitting on a table just at the side of me, and I was gently dunking the remote up and down into the tea. Margaret was terrified I could have electrocuted myself, but Geoff explained that you don't get much of a shock from a 12 volt system. Earlier I had been dunking my biscuits in my tea and must have got a bit confused.

Later, its night time, and Margaret and Geoff do the usual, they press the button to lower my bed and tuck me in. Geoff says 'goodnight Paddy' and Margaret, as she does each night, says 'goodnight, God bless, keep the light upon your chest.' The room is quiet and I close my eyes. Unfortunately, I'm not tired tonight, my mind is too active. I'm thinking of the past again and Dublin. It seems easy to remember my life from all those years ago, but I have trouble remembering yesterday. I drift a little, forcing myself to stay awake, but waiting for me in the dark are the shadows. There is a little light that glows in the corner of the room, a night light, but I still see the shadows. Across the room is my bathroom, and the door is slightly open. Someone is in there, dressed in black. A black shadow, and I know when I fall asleep he will come for me. I see vague outlines of people without faces. Are the people from my past here now? Are Nan, Molly and my mother telling me the tales of the shadows again, or am I dreaming? Have the shadows finally come to take me? I look at the bathroom door again and a shadow is moving in there. I want to shout to Margaret, but nothing comes out of my mouth. I know she will hear me, she is a very light sleeper and I have the baby alarm at the side of my bed. I try to reach for the alarm, but it falls onto the floor, so I reach across for the lamp at the side of the bed and switch it on.

Falling into a deep sleep I dream of the shadows. They are trying to smother me, and I can't breathe . . . Suddenly, I'm woken by the sound of Margaret's voice.

'Morning dad . . . oh my God, what have you been up to?' Margaret exclaims, wide eyed and confused. 'The baby alarm is on the floor and it's switched off . . . and what are you doing with a lamp across your chest. I'm surprised it hasn't burned your skin. Good job we're early risers or you might have shrivelled up.'

Margaret placed the lamp and the baby alarm back on the bedside table and switched the light off.

'The lamp is really hot Dad. It must have been on all night.'

She pressed the button on the bed that sits me up, and checks me over to see if I have burnt myself. I cannot speak yet to tell her about the shadows.

'I'll make you a nice cup of tea' she says 'best drink of the day, as you always say.' She puts a towel over my chest just like a napkin in readiness for me drinking the cup of tea and laughs, 'when I say "Goodnight, God Bless Keep the light Upon Your Chest" to you every night Dad. I don't mean it literally you know. You've just put a whole new meaning to that saying.'

Margaret walked off into the kitchen and I hear the kettle being filled with water. Soon she returns, and I sit up in bed drinking my cup of tea when I hear the door bell ring. Geoff shouts out, 'I'll get it' to Margaret. There is a discussion at the door and a few minutes later a nurse comes into my room, and once again I'm spoken to as if I am deaf or mentally retarded.

'Hello . . . Patrick, how are . . . you today. I've come to do a . . . depression test on you . . . this morning.'

A what? I'm not depressed.

'I just have to ask you a few questions about how you are feeling . . . to find out if you are depressed, it's just a procedure.'

Her face gets a little closer as she leans towards me, as if I hadn't heard her and she asks 'OKAY?'

I nod and the questions begin.

'Do you have little interest or pleasure in doing anything?'

Jaysus, now that's a question I can't answer, I don't understand it.

I nod my head, unsure why.

'Do you have trouble falling or staying asleep?'

How would I know I was falling, if I was asleep?

'Do you have trouble moving or speaking so slowly, other people could have noticed?

I say nothing.

'Or the opposite . . . do you feel so fidgety or restless, that you have been moving around a lot more than usual.'

Er what? Jaysus, I say nothing to that question. What the hell is she on about?

Geoff explains to the nurse that I cannot speak clearly enough to answer the questions. Even if I could speak clearly, I still couldn't answer the questions . . . I don't understand them. He see's my confusion and explains to the nurse how my Parkinson's affects my short term memory. Geoff answers the questions for me, and I nod my head when she asks me if that's right. Her last question was.

'Have you had any suicidal thoughts recently?'

Jaysus missis, I didn't until you came!! Fer God's sake, I'm forever fighting one ailment or another, would I be doing that if I felt suicidal. Jaysus, Mary, and Joseph, suicidal thoughts!

'That's good Patrick; you scored just one, which was, do you feel tired or have little energy.'

Geoff says to her.

'Well he is eighty four and does have Parkinson's disease. The medication makes him feel tired, but he doesn't sleep during the day. He enjoys reading the paper and still reads without needing glasses. We take him shopping, and he chooses his own clothes and he still goes on holiday, so I would say 'no' he doesn't get depressed.'

The nurse looked at me, I smile and she agrees with Geoff that I certainly don't appear to be depressed. The nurse says goodbye to me, inches from my face.

Jaysus, mother of God, I thought she was going to kiss me.

If possible, it's important to see the humorous sides of things, and luckily we've had plenty of laughs over the years. I remember one time when I was still sleeping upstairs and Margaret lost her mobile phone.

'Dad, have you seen my mobile phone? The last time it disappeared was when it was tucked down the side of your chair.'

'No I haven't seen it. Is it in the car?'

No. I looked. I can't find it anywhere and I've only just bought it.'

She searched the house for the phone. Cushions were pulled out and the furniture was lifted, but she couldn't find it anywhere. We were baffled. Margaret used the house phone to ring the mobile, but there was no sound from anywhere, and she assumed she must have lost it outside.

'It's certainly not in the house; I suppose I must have dropped it getting out of the car in town.'

'Is it upstairs?'

'No, I looked.'

That same night, while I was in bed, I heard this very loud 'Hello Moto' and jumped out of my skin. A phone then started ringing. The sound was coming from my laundry basket, which was stood in the corner of the room. I struggled to get out of bed and rummaged through my laundry. The phone was in my shirt pocket. The one I had worn the day before.

Over the years they have become used to finding things in my pockets; remote controls, sweets, and even half a sandwich once, not to mention anything I was given and disliked. Unknowingly, I tend to put things into the pockets of my trousers, shirts and even the pocket in my pyjama top. I had no idea what I was doing, and I was often asked if I had seen something they had lost. Antony's friend, Reece, came one day to work out in the gym at the bottom of the garden. When it was time to go home, he looked for his glasses and couldn't find them anywhere. Margaret asked if she could check my pockets and down the sides of my chair. It was a mystery because Reece said he had put them on the table where I had been sat at the time, and as far as he knew, they were still there when I moved to another chair.

'Dad, are you sure you haven't picked Reece's glasses up off the table?'

'No, I haven't seen them', I replied, turning to face Margaret.

Suddenly everyone was laughing. The glasses were on my face!

*

I heard Margaret and Geoff speaking very quietly somewhere in my room.

'He can't open his eyes again. I've tried waking him but he's not responding.'

'Oh no, not again' Margaret says, and I feel her near to the bed now. 'I don't think we should ring for a doctor yet though. We could wait to see if he opens them later like he did before. I think the panic in our voices scared him the last time.'

'I think you're right. I'll give him a wash and a shave, but we're going to have to try and give him his Parkinson's tablets; we can leave the rest of his tablets until later.'

I heard the sound of running water and Geoff gently touched my hand.

'I'm just going to give you a shave to make you feel better. I know you like to be clean and tidy. It's one of those silly days again when you have problems waking, but don't worry Paddy; it will pass as it always does. We're here with you. You're not on your own, and you're in your own bed at home.'

I felt frustrated and wondered why I couldn't open my eyes, yet, I could hear. What does he mean? *"It's one of those silly days again, when you having problems waking."* Has this happened before? Short term memory is what they tell me, so does this mean I will be able to remember this day in the future. When Geoff began washing my face I became aware of Margaret's voice.

'Come on Dad; try to open your eyes, wakey, wakey.'

They must have got used to this occurrence by now, because they left me to rest, but not until they had given me my medication.

180

'I'm going to raise the bed slowly Paddy and give you a sip of water to moisten your mouth, and then we're going to try and give you these two tablets.'

I felt the tilt of the bed, and Geoff gave me a sip of water, which took me by surprise and I coughed. On the second attempt I managed to drink quite a few mouthfuls before the tablets were put on my tongue, and I was lowered back down. Suddenly, as if nothing had happened at all, my eyes opened and I was awake.

'It's about time' Margaret gasped 'You've been asleep all day. We were just about to ring the doctor.'

All day!

'I'm hungry.' I said in a whisper.

She laughed. 'The day you lose your appetite, will be the day I really will start to worry.

A nursing sister came to change my catheter a few days later, and Geoff was telling her about the long sleeps I have and the days I can hear, but I am unable to open my eyes.

'You're better off letting him sleep, so long as he's all right when he does wake up. If his voice is slurred or his face has fallen to one side, then ring for an ambulance without delay. But it could just be his body that's healing itself, so try to make sure he drinks plenty of water if you can.'

'He does manage to sip water' Margaret said 'so we can still give him his main tablets, but it's strange that he can't open his eyes, yet at certain times he can respond. I think most of the time he is sleeping and not aware of what is happening. Whatever it is doesn't seem to distress him, although it did upset him the first time it happened.'

'It could be a mini stroke that he's having.' The nurse explained 'what we call a TIA, a Transient Ischaemic Attack. It's caused by a temporary disruption in the blood supply to a part of the brain.'

'Is it serious'? Margaret asked.

'Well, the disruption in blood supply can cause symptoms similar to those of a stroke, such as speech or visual disturbance, and numbness or weakness in the arms and legs. However, a TIA does not last as long a stroke. The effects sometimes only last for a few minutes and are usually fully resolved within 24 hours. The problem is that it could be his Parkinson's that's at the bottom of these prolonged sleeps. We really don't know. Make sure he has plenty of sips of water if you can get him to swallow, and just try to give him his main medication for Parkinson's if you can. Keep him comfortable and if you're concerned, phone your GP.'

Margaret mentioned it was eleven years since I was diagnosed with Parkinson's, and how I had probably had the disease for a while before then. I thought of all the changes that have occurred over these last few years. They may be minor things, like my staring into space for long periods without blinking, leaving my eyes dry and sore. Or how my face seems to have gradually lost a lot of its expressions, and how finding it hard to smile, makes it hard to show my feelings. Sometimes I watch spiders weaving webs when everyone else is oblivious to them, and I see children in the garden and wave to them when I know in my heart they're not there. I don't really have trouble getting off to sleep, but I wake up every few hours and very often remember my terrible dreams.

The district nurse smiled at me and said comfortingly.

'I'm sure you will be alright Patrick. I don't think it's anything to worry about too much. I've finished changing your catheter, so I will be back in about three months. It's always a pleasure to come and see you.'

I waved back to her and did my best to smile back. I have to say that even though the catheter change is now a lot easier; the district nurses were still just as gentle and considerate, and tried hard to keep my self-respect.

Before my illness I used to love to sing along to music, and Margaret still encourages me to sing now by playing familiar music I once loved to hear. When she bought the film 'Abba the Movie', she had me waving my hands in the air and clapping along to the songs. We would watch it time and time again, and use the music to help me do exercises and keep my muscles supple. It was Margaret's way of attempting to stop my joints from becoming stiff. One day while the film was playing, I felt strangely tense and rigid. My head wouldn't stay still. It was moving in circles, round and round and I could only focus on the ceiling. My whole head felt like a bag of sawdust and I was shaking violently. I felt as though I was twisting inside and I cried out in an unusually loud voice.

'What's happening to my body? Help me!'

Margaret and Geoff tried to calm me down and I could see they were as frightened as I was. After a little while I began to respond to their calming influences, and I didn't feel as scared as I had when the episode first started. Both of them were reassuring me that I would be alright, and that it was only my medication which was causing these strange sensations. Geoff commented he had noticed how, just after taking my tablets, I had begun to rotate my head, open my mouth and start to stare at the ceiling and said to Margaret.

'I've been thinking about this.' He said to Margaret. 'I think he is over medicated now. These episodes of vagueness only seem to happen after his lunchtime, teatime and suppertime tablets. He's perfectly fine on a morning, and I've noticed he's at his worst around tea time. I wonder if it has anything to do with the time difference between the late evening and morning tablets. Perhaps later in the day he's getting the dosage too close together, or perhaps he doesn't need as much medication as he used to. There's no sign of shaking or stiffness in a morning either and that's the longest gap between taking his tablets. We're due to see the specialist at the hospital next month, so I'll telephone the Parkinson's liaison nurse, and ask if we can take out the teatime tablet, and space out the others.'

'Good idea.' She replied, holing my hand. 'And that will give us a few weeks to monitor what's happening to him. Something's not right.'

After discussions with the liaison nurse, it was decided they should reduce my medication by twenty five percent, and monitor any effects this might have before reporting the results to the specialist. After about a week of taking one tablet when I woke up, and one late in the afternoon, followed by one just before I when to sleep, the head movements stopped. I didn't stare vaguely at the ceiling with my mouth open anymore, and I felt much brighter and could make myself understood more easily.

When we went to see the specialist, he asked if there had been any new developments. Geoff explained about the vagueness, and how they had reduced the medication and monitored my reactions. The specialist agreed that after a while the effectiveness of the medication can wear off, or the need for it can reduce, and that making the changes had obviously been beneficial. After checking me over as usual, and asking me a few questions about how I was feeling, he said he would write to our GP to confirm the new dosage and would see us again in six months.

That had been quite straight forward and easy to arrange, but on the other hand, some things prove more difficult to sort out. I still had my own teeth, but as with older people, my gums were receding and one tooth had worked its way loose. It was very difficult, in fact almost impossible, for me to chew anything, and we were all worried I might swallow the tooth whilst eating or worse still, while I was asleep. I could easily have choked on the tooth. We needed a dentist. No problem you would think, but the dentist I was registered with had an upstairs surgery, and of course there was no way we could get up the stairs. Margaret rang around the other dental surgeries in our area, but none of the NHS dentists that were taking new patients had wheelchair access. She rang our doctor's surgery, who said they couldn't help as it was a dental problem. She rang the local hospital, but they said I would have to be referred.

No one appeared to be able to refer me, and by this time things were getting desperate. By chance, Geoff heard of a NHS clinic that specialised in many medical fields, including dentistry, and it was situated at ground level. You would think the problem was solved, but we still needed a referral. Geoff rang our Parkinson's liaison nurse, but she was on holiday for a couple of weeks. In desperation, he rang the clinic and explained the situation. The lady on reception was very sympathetic and told him.

'As Patrick's official primary carer, you can refer him yourself.'

'Consider him referred,' Geoff told her, 'when can we come in? Things are really desperate.'

The following day, I was sat in my wheelchair, with a plastic gown draped around me, and the dentist was busily extracting the tooth, which had been giving us all so many problems.

*

One of my earliest memories of Parkinson's disease was that I wasn't swallowing my saliva properly, and I seemed be making more than usual. At first, I was able to carry a handkerchief, and no one noticed. Now, years later, it was becoming a big problem because I wasn't swallowing my saliva in a normal way, and my chin was very sore and chapped. Unfortunately, the saliva sometimes goes into my lungs, and I get frequent chest infections and even pneumonia as a result of this. Geoff explained this to my consultant at the Parkinson's clinic, and he said if I was willing to try it, he had a cure. It was called Botox.

An appointment was made for me to go to a special clinic, and Geoff took me there in the Pope Mobile. When I had my first injections, the needle was painfully pushed through my cheeks and neck, into my saliva glands. Within a week the Botox worked, it tightened up my saliva glands and I stopped dribbling. Of course, I was teased about it at home, and told how much younger and handsome I looked. I've had quite a few of these injections, and most of them have worked well, although after one session, I had more saliva than ever, and it constantly trickled down my throat, causing me to cough. The saliva collected in my throat and I coughed all night long. Geoff tried to encourage me to cough it up into a tissue, but I hadn't the energy to do it, I was too tired and exhausted. For weeks the cough continued. I had antibiotics twice, but it didn't clear up, and we were all shattered from lack of sleep.

The hospital where I have the Botox injections made an appointment for a month's time to try again, but in the meantime I knew I was ill. The doctor was called. I remember Margaret holding my hand and crying, and I was aware of the locum doctor speaking to them. I heard him say to Margaret and Geoff that I was very poorly, and he comforted Margaret as she was crying uncontrollably. It was all very emotional and I wondered if both Margaret and Geoff believed this was the end. Was I dying? Geoff was asking the doctor questions and I knew that he was as upset as Margaret. I could tell from his voice. The doctor made a phone call outside in the garden, and soon the ambulance arrived. The paramedics lifted me onto a trolley and Margaret wrapped me up in blankets, long before they got a chance to. Apparently, I was to be taken straight onto a ward and did not have to go through casualty. The doctor had sorted it all out on the telephone. He didn't want me to spend hours waiting on a trolley. I remember very little of being in hospital, but I knew that Geoff stayed with me all the time I was in there, sleeping on a recliner chair at the side of me. The reason he stayed the night was because, being unable to speak for myself, he liked to be around when a doctor came to see me. He knew I would probably become confused and unknowingly, I would pull the intravenous drips out of my arm, and anything else that was attached to me, as I had done in the past. After only three days on intravenous drips, I was to shock the hospital staff and my family once more. I started to recover. This was all thanks to the medical staff at the hospital, and of course Geoff staying to ensure I received my Parkinson's medication on the dot. All I had to do now was to get my strength back.

A young ward doctor came to see me one evening while Geoff had gone for something to eat. Margaret was with me at the time. The doctor asked some questions and one of them was.

'Does he suffer from dementia?'

No, I do not suffer from dementia. Thank you very much. I am well aware of what you're saying!

I know people think I must suffer from dementia, simply because I cannot always speak. If I could converse with them, I would say.

'My vocal cords may not work, but my brain does.'

186

Thankfully Margaret said. 'No, he doesn't have dementia. He has problems with his vocal cords.'

The doctor then asked me to stick my tongue out for him; I refused to do it. I was expected to drink plenty of fluids, and when Margaret tried to give me a drink of water I wouldn't drink it. Earlier, Geoff had to feed me because I wouldn't hold the cutlery, and when the tea lady brought me a cup of tea, I refused to drink out of the hospital cup that had a spout; waiting until the lid was taken off. I sulked when Margaret and Geoff went for a coffee together, because I couldn't go with them, and I wouldn't respond to them when they came back. I was acting like a naughty child again. Being stubborn was one of the things I was still good at, and I know I was being unreasonable, but I wanted to go home. I had no other means of complaining.

When the medication had taken control of the infection, I was told I might be allowed to recover in my own bed at home. That was if I could show them I could stand and walk a few steps. As soon as the consultant left the small ward I was in, Geoff swung me onto the edge of the bed and put my slippers on for me. Clipping my catheter bag onto a walking frame, he helped me to stand, and I walked into the hospital corridor just as my consultant came out of the next ward. The doctor smiled at me and nodded.

'You can go home now Mr Millar.'

Oh, I was so pleased to be home. There was always that deep down fear in my mind of going into the rehabilitation hospital again. The following morning the sun shone in my room, and there was the sound of the kettle boiling and breakfast cooking. I had cereals, followed by scrambled egg for my breakfast, and I didn't need to be spoon fed.

*

Margaret and Geoff had decided it would be better if Geoff stayed with me when I was admitted to hospital. I was having difficulty in communicating with the doctors and the nursing staff. It wasn't so much as I didn't know what I was suffering from; it was just my short term memory that was not functioning properly.

I knew I had Parkinson's disease. I also knew I was suffering from a chest infection, and clearly understood I was on medication for these ailments, but unfortunately, I just could not relate one thing to another, or put them in any kind of time scale. Basically, Parkinson's left me confused and I would react in two ways. I would make out I didn't know, or I would simply agree to whatever the medical staff wanted to hear. To illustrate this, there were more than a few occasions when I was asked if smoked. My response would be that I had given up some months, or at best a few years ago, when in fact I hadn't smoked for over forty years.

Not being able to relate time scales with symptoms, or indeed not being able to associate daily occurrences as being symptoms, would have put me at risk of being wrongly diagnosed and could have placed a considerable burden on the doctors and nurses. The doctors would have had a hard job of working out what was wrong with me, and the nurses would have no idea what my individual needs were when they were trying to make me comfortable. Little wonder Margaret and Geoff were so frustrated by the obstacles and reasons that were put forward when it was suggested Geoff should stay with me. Over my first few instances of being admitted onto a ward, Geoff was told that it was against hospital policy . . . there was nowhere for him to sleep. . . every other patient's relatives would want to stay. . . or that it just wasn't necessary. After showing great determination, and a refusal to leave me on my own, Geoff was allowed to stay, sleeping on an easy chair at my bedside. Mostly, when the doctors had been supplied with all the information they required, and after Geoff had helped me to wash, shave and make the most of my mealtimes, it was usually accepted that it was better if he stayed; most times, though not always.

Another reason for Geoff's insistence on staying with me was to make sure I received my Parkinson's medication on time. Of course, a busy medical ward needs to have a system when it comes to distributing patient's medication. There are usually set times when the medicine trolley is wheeled around the ward and everyone are given their tablets, or other types of medication, but this method doesn't work if your tablet regime is completely designed to suit your individual needs; as in the case of

188

Parkinson's disease. It is not possible for a nurse to remember just which hour a tablet, or series of tablets, need to be taken; but a person who looks after someone with Parkinson's does know. Geoff knew exactly when each batch of tablets needed to be taken, and half an hour before they were due, he would quietly remind the nurses, giving them time to make the necessary arrangements.

Some of the staff really appreciated Geoff being there to help out with the mundane daily tasks. This took the pressure off of them with regard to tablet times, mealtime feeding, and even letting him on occasions take me for a bath. None the less, he needed to be as diplomatic as possible. Despite the hospital matron having run a campaign about Parkinson's disease awareness, some of the medical staff resented his presence, and one particular nurse made this abundantly clear. After repeatedly being asked to give me my medication when I needed to take it, the male nurse in question made us wait until the normal rounds time, setting off in the opposite direction around the ward, to the other staff. Apart from my tablets being well overdue to start with, I was now the last one the nurse came to, adding another thirty minutes to the time I had to wait.

Geoff insisted that it was worth the inconvenience of staying with me to help the nurses in any way he could, and to ensure that I didn't pull out my cannula and the tubes for my drip. Of course Margaret, and other members of the family, came during visiting times, and throughout the night Geoff was able to sleep next to my bed, which made me feel more secure and less confused. Often, I would wake up during the night, wide awake and gently folding my bed sheet over my chest. Geoff knew that I was content and felt secure.

Chapter Twelve

Return of the Shadow Men

(2011/2012)

Even now, after all these years, Margaret kindly bullies me into fighting this disease. She tries to make sure I exercise both my body and my mind, and she will ask me questions now and again.

'Dad, what's your date of birth?'

I tell her, and she asks me what our house number is. Which street do we live in? What was the name of the army barracks I'd been posted to? These memories seemed to be locked in my brain, and up to a few years ago I could even remember my National Insurance Number. She never gives up. I watch old programmes that make me laugh, 'to exercise my face,' and we sit in the conservatory listening to 1950s music as well as Irish music. I try hard to sing along to help strengthen my vocal cords, and enjoy myself.

Geoff always makes sure I am taken to the toilet twice a day, every day, to try to open my bowels. It doesn't matter what is happening at the time or who is in the house. To give me privacy I have a whistle to blow when I've finished. Neither of them is prepared to let me give in to the illness, and I am told continually by everyone how well I look. I am never made to feel a burden to either of them, and woe betides anyone who doesn't treat me with respect. We do everything together, and we make the most of every day and situation, even though we never know just what the outcome will be.

'Do you feel like going for a walk around that lovely nature reserve with the big lake, the one near Wakefield, Paddy?' One day Geoff asked, already bringing the wheelchair towards me. 'It'll make a nice change from sitting in the garden. We can call for a glass of Guinness on the way home and sit in the beer garden. Bonny can come with us, then she can have a swim in the lake, she'll love that.'

I nodded my head, but I didn't feel very good. I was weak and my body ached, I was leaning to the left again, and my upper body sat on my hips unsupported. Floppy is the word I'm looking for.

I felt floppy.

The scenery was nice and the weather was just right, not too hot or windy, but seeing young people running around the lake, glancing down on me, left me feeling sad. I could see the sympathy in their eyes. They see a shrivelled up old man in a wheelchair leaning to the left, with his head drooping, I hadn't the strength to hold it in place. Oh, to be able to walk among people again, to run and kick a ball with my family, just one more time before I die. I watch Margaret and Nicholas throwing sticks for Bonny to fetch back, and I remember a time when we went to the lake long ago. Bonny had come out of the water with a huge fish in her mouth, and as usual in these circumstances, the camera wasn't at hand and the fish wriggled free. My thoughts were broken when Geoff stopped to give me a drink of water from a bottle. I was having trouble holding my head up, and the liquid dribbled down my shirt. We walked until we had completed the circle all the way around the lake, which they tell me is roughly a two mile walk, and on the way home, as promised, we stopped for a drink outside the nearest pub. Geoff brought me a glass of Guinness, but I couldn't lift my head up to drink without it spilling and I felt like crying.

When we arrived home, Geoff put me to bed, I was too weak to shuffle to the top of the bed, and Nicholas gave Geoff a hand to lift me onto the pillows. Nicholas stayed with me and talked about the walk we had just been on. I kept my eyes down and whispered to him.

'I'm sorry for spoiling it for you all.'

'Don't be silly Granddad, it isn't your fault. You have times like this but you always bounce back.'

We talked a little more about our trip, and I wondered how Nicholas felt seeing his great grandfather like this. He will never know the real person and what I was like when I was active. When he was younger I never had the chance to play football with him, as I had done with his father so many times. Nicholas is eighteen now and often sits and talks to me, waiting patiently for me to speak about my life in the forces, and the times I spent with my best friend Ralph.

'I was thinking of joining the forces. Do you think I should, Granddad?'

'Yes, you should.'

'Did you enjoy it when you were in the army?'

'No.'

Nicholas laughed so hard, and so did I. He laughed even more when I suddenly started shadow boxing.

'What are you trying to say?' Nicholas laughed 'that you did a lot of fighting?'

I nodded my head, laughing, remembering when I was a youngster.

Living in the heart of Dublin City, there were street gangs just as there probably are today. Every district of Dublin had its own gang, but the worst gang of all, was known as the Animal Gang. No one would dare to fight with them. They didn't fist fight like the rest of us; the Animal Gang used blades which were in the peaks of their caps, and would lash out with their caps, slashing anyone who crossed their path. This put many people in hospital, and Nicholas would have laughed if I could have told him how people were carted off to hospital in prams, regardless of their age and size. It wasn't a case of phoning for an ambulance in those days, people were rushed there by any means possible.

It's very hard for me to get out what I want to say, and it can take a while for me to explain what I am thinking about. It's a pleasure to remember things, and share them with someone who is prepared to spend the time it takes for me to make myself understood. Nicholas always waits patiently for me to tell my story, he will sit at the side of my chair, or bed, until I am finished, and he laughs when I tell him funny things about my childhood.

When I was all tucked up, Margaret comes in to see me.

'Dad, I know you were feeling out of sorts today at the lake, but you should never think you're spoiling anything. We're a family. Remember when we used to say we were the three musketeers, all for one and one for all. Well that's still the case and we do all right. We're a team. Don't ever consider yourself a burden. We don't think that, and we never will. It isn't your fault you have an illness like this, it's that blooming Mr Parkinson's fault,' she laughed, 'anyway, Geoff's going to phone the doctor in the morning and get a prescription. We think you have a water infection. It's the first one you have had for a long time, and when it's better we're going on a trip to Cambridge. We have all sorts of plans for day trips this summer.'

She kisses the top of my head and I feel so much better now. Geoff comes back into the room and he also reassures me.

'It's just another hiccup and hiccups soon pass.'

And it did, I was well again in no time, and as promised we went out visiting places. Because both Nicholas and Antony, his younger brother live with us now, they are a great help to Margaret and Geoff, and they often come with us on our day trips and help by taking it in turns to push my wheelchair. It never occurred to me when I was an able man, the difficulties of being disabled. Take for example when we visited a few museums in North Yorkshire only to find the corridors were too narrow for a wheelchair. The rooms were very tiny and it was difficult to manoeuvre, or to be able to turn into the doorways, especially in the workhouse and prison museums. Even though a lift had been installed to get us from one floor to another, I didn't see much, as these places were very small and tight. I suppose there isn't much that can be changed in places such as these to adapt to wheelchair access, although they certainly do their best. The whole point is to keep everything as it was to retain the authenticity.

Now, before setting off anywhere, we have to make sure it's wheelchair friendly. Probably one of the worst experiences of all, for people in wheelchairs, is the dropped kerbs that are not flush with the road. Crossing from one pavement to another at side streets, can feel like a game of Russian roulette as cars came from both right and the left. I always feel as if I'm about to be thrown out of the chair as it bumps down onto the road, and as well as that, I'm tipped backwards as we try to negotiate the step at the other side. I feel deeply for younger disabled people. I've had my days travelling and going to different places. I have a modern wheelchair now, with wings on the side to prevent me leaning to the left, and an adjustable headrest and deep cushions. There are brakes on the handlebars as well as at the side of me, and after the episode with Margaret going downhill and being unable to stop, this makes me feel more secure. It was thanks to the mobile physiotherapist I have a wheelchair with such comfort. He said a standard wheelchair was not suitable for me, especially when I leaned to the left, and suggested we should call in the occupational therapist, informing her that he insisted we have a custom made chair.

I have good days and I have bad days. Unfortunately, now the bad days are overtaking the good days, and occasionally, I feel really down. I want to be able to join in conversations with my family when I hear them talking, and find it frustrating when I can't have my say. Being unable to join in a conversation is probably, for me, the hardest part of Parkinson's to accept. On a good day I find I can talk more easily, and providing I am given time to get the words out, I can explain myself very well, but more and more, I hear everyone talking around me and I can't join in. So many times I have wanted to say something, but before I can get just one little word out, the conversation has moved on. Not that anyone seems to understand me much, apart from Margaret and Geoff. I suppose after living together for over ten years they have learned to understand me better than anyone. But now as the years have gone by and my Parkinson's has developed I struggle to make myself heard. The change in your speech is a very slow progression. The process happens over such a long period of time that it's not until someone else notices a dramatic change that you realise how much your ability to communicate has been lost. Unfortunately, by this time it is generally too late to do anything about it.

I want to do the things I remember. I want to walk up and down the garden again and take Bonny into the field, and I long to shower and dress myself. I remember these things, but my short term memory is not very efficient and I can't recall daily events. When it comes to remembering memories from the past, that's a different thing, it's as if they happened only yesterday and I remember them very well. So I have the one thing that is precious to me, whether it's a good day or a bad day, and that's memories of my life. Geoff once said to me.

'Don't worry that you have short term memory loss, Paddy. Margaret and I will be your memory. No-one can take away the memories you have stored away in your mind; memories of Joyce and your family. They're much more important than memories of today.'

Parkinson's has taken away my ability to remember what's happening at the present time. Some of the time I don't know what day or even what month or year it is, but I do understand some things. For example, if I am told we are going somewhere tomorrow, or that it's a special day. I will often wake up early on that particular morning and be looking forward to it. I may have to be reminded about what's actually going to happen, but I know something is going on and I'm eager to join in. It's a strange thing, but these events that are unclear in my short term memory sometimes reappear at a later date. Perhaps they have become a different kind of memory.

Most of my faculties are still intact and I can still join in and enjoy a joke. I watch TV programmes where they make fun of what is happening in the world, and love to watch Question Time. I used to watch it with Joyce, and when Question time is on now, I try to stay awake until it's finished; listening to what they have to say and wanting to join in. Films and long drama programmes do present a problem, as I find difficulty in remembering the plot, my mind drifting off into other directions. When my attention is brought back to the screen, I have usually forgotten what is happening.

Unbelievably, I have somehow got used to pain over the years, and it's probably because I don't know what to expect anymore, having no recollection of what it felt like the first time. I regularly get praised for sitting quietly while a needle is inserted into my arm, or into my saliva glands, when having Botox treatment. However, one morning the doorbell chimed and a nurse came dashing through the door to my room. There was no 'Good morning Patrick' as all the nursing staff call out, or any signs of communication from her, other than to tell Geoff she was here to do a suprapubic catheter change. Normally, the procedure takes anything up to thirty minutes while the nurse takes the catheter out very slowly. The surrounding area is cleaned with sterile water and a new catheter is carefully inserted into my abdomen. There is usually a slight discomfort, but not nearly as painful as it used to be in the past. In those days, not only was it tremendously painful, but it was also extremely embarrassing having a young nurse, young enough to be my great granddaughter, do the procedure. Indeed, in all the years of having my catheter changed, male nurses have seemed to be few and far between.

This particular morning, the nurse, without prior warning, pulled the tube out in one almighty tug. I almost jumped off the bed with the shock and pain. Geoff had only gone to the medicine cupboard for the sterile water. As he walked back through the door, the nurse was already pushing the new catheter in with so much force that I screamed out. Then she was gone, leaving me and Geoff in disbelief at the speed of her coming and going. I don't remember much of the following weeks, though I do remember being unable to stand up because of the pain. Apparently, I was pale, weak and unaware of my surroundings. I was told later, that the following day I slept for eighteen hours and instead of waking up and being my normal self; I had a very high temperature, and was unable to sip water or take my medication. Once again, Margaret was forced to phone the emergency doctor as it was out of surgery hours. She explained my symptoms and told the doctor about the nurse and my catheter change.

'He hasn't been right since. He's really spaced out and very hot. We've have never known him like this before, other than when he has pneumonia. He doesn't have a cough and his breathing isn't laboured, so I don't think it's his chest. The nurse didn't clean the area before she inserted the new catheter. We're convinced he has an infection.'

Within half an hour the doctor came out to see me. I had seen this particular doctor before and he remembered me. He was very pleasant and unrushed, taking his time to thoroughly examine me. He was convinced it was indeed a urine infection.

'The nurse may have pushed bacteria from the skin around the site directly into his bladder. I agree with you,' he said to Margaret. 'She should have cleaned the surrounding area first, as scabs do sometimes form. I'll give him some antibiotics, and if you feel he's getting any worse tonight, don't hesitate to call me. I would inform your GP first thing tomorrow about the nurse's behaviour.'

I have to say that the medical care and amount of help and assistance we've received from our local medical centre has been second to none. We never had any cause to feel dissatisfied or complain, but the behaviour of this nurse needed reporting, and when the doctor had left, Geoff wrote a letter explaining the treatment I had received. The next morning he took two copies up to the surgery, one for our GP and one for the nursing team. Within hours, the head of the district nursing team came down to apologise for the nurse's negligence. He told us she had been reprimanded, and would have to go on a re-training course. Geoff and Margaret were much more interested in how my condition was deteriorating. For almost twenty four hours I had been sleeping, unable to eat anything and giving my medication was extremely difficult. It seems that I remained like this for the best part of three days. Geoff went back to giving me my medication in small spoonfuls of custard, as he had done in the hospital; but crushing

197

the tablets means they don't work as well. When this was added to the fact that as I was not able to eat anything substantial, my condition began to spiral downwards and our GP came to see me. She was concerned the nurse could have ruptured my bladder when inserting the catheter. Luckily, on inspection, she was convinced this was not the case, but she was still worried about the infection, and took a sample of my urine. It was tested in the laboratory to find the correct strain of infection, enabling the doctor to give me the appropriate medication. Very soon after taking the new antibiotic, I was beginning to feel better, but was still too weak to stand. It was now over two weeks since the catheter change. Now I was confined to bed and unable to do the exercises that would prevent my muscles from locking. The weakness was beginning to have a bad effect on my body. Geoff and Margaret could do nothing but watch as I began to waste away.

None of these recent problems had anything to do with Parkinson's disease. They were the direct result of my not being able to get out of bed, and being so weak opened the door for another problem to start. My swallowing had been slightly affected by Parkinson's from the onset, but mostly I had always been strong enough to swallow or cough any moisture away. Now, because I didn't have the strength to cough, little by little, the saliva I was making, along with small amounts of the fluids I was drinking, were running down the back of my throat and into my lungs. I was beginning to aspirate and the fluid became infected. At first, every effort was made to keep me out of hospital, but we realised the antibiotics were no longer helping and we had to recognise defeat and I was admitted to a ward by the doctor.

Since sleeping on an air mattress at home, there had been virtually no problems with pressure sores on my heels, and only very occasionally on my bottom. Geoff was very insistent as soon as we arrived at the hospital, on how urgently I needed a pressure relief mattress. He showed the nursing staff the tenderness around my heels, and how obvious it was from the discoloured skin that I had suffered from pressure sores before. The nurse who admitted me telephoned the stores for a mattress, but we waited in vain.

The doctors and nurses very quickly installed a cannula and started to feed me with antibiotic drips and saline to fight the chest infection, and replace lost fluids. Geoff arranged to stay to help care and also speak for me. Everything was being done, apart from the special mattress. Geoff kept stressing to the nursing staff how severe the bed sores were previously, and how important it was to prevent the same thing happening again. From my previous stays in hospital, we knew it could be many hours before an air bed was brought up from the bedding store, but we were told repeatedly there wasn't a mattress available.

Apparently pressure ulcers can develop very quickly in people who are at high risk, and it can take less than an hour for an ulcer to develop. Very soon we could literally see the pressure sores begin to form. First they were Grade 1 sores, where the skin is permanently red, feels warm and slightly swollen, but has not yet broken. Then quickly they moved on to Grade 2, where the ulcer, though still superficial, looks like a blister or abrasion. Both Geoff and Margaret were becoming frantic, and kept asking for an air mattress, but still there wasn't one available. We couldn't really blame the nursing staff, they were doing their best. Pillows were placed under my heels to try to absorb the pressure, something we never had to do at home, but it was too late, the damage had been done. The blisters on my heels had reached Grade 3. There was damage to the tissues underneath the skin, and to make matters worse, there were sores appearing on my bottom.

Thankfully, the antibiotic drips were getting to grips with the chest infection, and after a couple of days I was showing signs of my old self. It's quite remarkable how quickly these antibiotic drips work, and I was determined to get back home. Soon, I was discharged and it was arranged that the district nurses would see to my needs.

Unfortunately after some blood tests were taken, we had a phone call from our GP to say I had to go back into hospital. The results had shown abnormalities in my sodium levels. It was approximately three in the afternoon when we arrived, and again, Geoff immediately asked the nurse if she could arrange an air mattress, explaining what had happened a few days ago, and she reassured us she would see to it as soon as she had completed the admittance procedure.

After waiting a further six hours and constantly inquiring about an air bed, we were still being told they would see to one for me. At 11:00 pm, Geoff and Margaret went to the nurses' station to complain about how we were being ignored. They explained that we understood the nurses were busy, and were obviously short of beds and staff, but Geoff stressed how urgently I needed an air bed. Apart from a sympathetic agreement that things could be better, once again, nothing happened. By midnight Geoff and Margaret were extremely annoyed, I wasn't even wearing a wrist band, nor had I been assessed, and they realised I probably hadn't even been fully admitted onto the ward. I certainly hadn't seen a doctor . . . and was still lying on a standard hospital mattress. Geoff went back to the nurses' station, and because the nursing staff had changed over, the night shift received the full force of Geoff's anger. Over an hour later a doctor finally appeared at the side of my bed, and after checking me over, he took some blood samples and informed us the results would be known the following day. It was now nearly two in the morning, both Geoff and Margaret were both extremely tired. I was drifting off to sleep and as I didn't need any more Parkinson's tablets until the morning; they decided to go home and get some rest.

Early the following day, they were back to make sure I was receiving my medication on time. There was still no sign of a pressure relief mattress, but at least I had slept reasonably well and was in good spirits. During the morning the results of the blood test came back and, along with the intravenous drip, and all the water I had been encouraged to drink, the doctor said I could be discharged.

Transferring me from the bed to my wheelchair was extremely hard and the pain must have shown on my face. The pressure sores were now Grade 4, the most severe form. The ulcers were deep, and there was damage to the muscle and possibly the bone underneath.

As soon as we had arrived home from the hospital, Geoff had telephoned the leader of our district nursing team to explain the extent of my pressure sores. The head nurse agreed to come straight round to do an assessment. He was appalled by the state of my heels and the sores on my bottom, insisting he needed to make out a special report. He measured the size of the wounds, which were now completely open and ulcerated, then filled in the report, and using some of the dressings we had left over from the last time, he made me as comfortable as possible. He then wrote out a long list of supplies to pick up from the chemist shop.

When Geoff went to the Pharmacy to pick up the prescription, he purposely asked the Pharmacist, who we had know for quite some time, how much the big cardboard box full of dressing, creams and ointments would cost the NHS. He was shocked to hear the contents were worth in excess of £500. It seemed ridiculous to all of us that this expense, plus the cost of the district nurses coming, sometimes two at a time, should all be wasted, when a pressure relief mattress and a pump only cost roughly the same £500. It can't be cheap to send a district nurse three times a week. We had begged the hospital staff to supple an air mattress. Surely, in the long run, thousands of pounds could be saved on medications, dressings, nurses and doctors visits, if the hospital had a good supply of air beds for the elderly and infirm. After all, from much experience I know they work in preventing bedsores.

The leader of the district nurses made arrangements for a team of specialists to come to the house and confirm that the procedures he was following would indeed combat the severity of my wounds. All three of the members of this team were shocked at the way in which I had been discharged with severe pressure sores; as indeed was one of our own GPs, who, when he came to visit, just stood and shook his head in disbelief.

On one of his many visits to check on my progress, I was listening to our local head district nurse telling Geoff and Margaret how they sometimes have to use maggot therapy if there is no improvement. The nurse was explaining how maggots eat the rotting flesh and how they can work well with pressure sores. On hearing this, I was shocked to say the least. Margaret, realising I was listening and becoming distressed, quickly said that they weren't real maggots they used, and it was just a treatment they termed as 'Maggots'. I knew they were talking about real ones. I had watched a film once where a man fell from a cliff and lay there for days as the wound on his leg festered. The maggots had eaten all the rotting flesh, thus preventing Gangrene setting in, and he survived. The treatment obviously works, but still, I didn't relish the idea of maggots crawling all over my foot.

Would I be able to feel them eating my flesh?

A new district nurse, we hadn't seen before, came to change my dressings one morning. She stayed awhile, talking to Margaret and me, telling us about when she had been a nurse in the army a good few years ago.

'Pressure sore were very rare when I was a young nurse. I was trained to give a good bed bath every morning for those who were unable to take a bath. We were taught how to massage each part of the patient's body with a flannel, to aide circulation, and we made sure our patients were turned to different positions throughout the day. This stopped them from getting sores in the first place. Of course, the matron was always nearby to make sure the patients were given everything they needed to make their stay in hospital comfortable, including encouraging them to eat and drink.'

When I returned from that short stay in hospital, I knew I was going to be confined to my bed for a long time, if not forever. I'm much older now. I was told the district nurse would have to come three times a week to change my dressings and replace them with new ones. I overheard the nurse telling Margaret and Geoff that repairing the dead flesh on my heel would take a lot more work using special dressings; often changing the type of medication that goes onto the sore itself, until the wound gradually starts to heal. Being bed bound would only make matters worse. The longer I stayed in bed, the less I would be using my leg muscles, and very quickly they would start to waste away. Unless I could exercise my

202

legs or the pressure sores could heal, I would once again be the victim of the same vicious circle.

*

Bonny has died and I miss her. When I'm alone, I weep for her, just as they all try to hide their tears from me. Nicholas and Antony, who have lived with us a few years now, avoid coming into my room for fear of upsetting me. Margaret's eyes are puffy and I hear Antony, who's bedroom is above mine, sobbing. For all this time Bonny has slept in my room, watching over me, sometimes casually resting her head on the bed and looking into my eyes. My room isn't the same without her gentle breathing. I always knew one of us would have to be the first to go, and I also knew she would have grieved for me as I do for her. I close my eyes and think of all the years I was lucky to have shared with Bonny, her protectiveness, whenever a dog raced towards us when out walking, her frantic bark whenever I fell, and the way she lay beside me resting her chin on my chest. Bonny arrived the year Joyce died and has always been good company, from my long stays at Margaret's to her moving here. Without her I doubt very much I would have walked around the playing field each day for all those years. Whichever chair I was sat in Bonny was beside me, or straight opposite me, where she could keep an eye on my every movement. The nights are very lonely without her, and I feel frightened now. I knew I was safe from the Shadows, but without her to protect me, I feel they are closing in and I know it won't be long before I join her.

Night time has always been the worst time of all. I hardly sleep. Listening to the baby alarm upstairs, Margaret told me she could hear me talking to someone, and had come downstairs to see if I was all right. Of course, I was wide awake.

'I can't believe you're still awake. I could hear you talking. It must be a long night for you, not being able to sleep, would you like the television on for company.'

I nodded my head.

'I'm going to have to turn the sound down really low, or it'll keep me awake, is that okay?'

I nod again and she kisses me on the forehead and leaves the room. Sometimes when I do sleep, I wake up and try to open my eyes and I can't. I can't move. And when I eventually do manage to open my eyes, the black shadows are back, waiting for me in the corner of the room. I can see the hooded figures walking my way, ready to hold me down. One of the cloaked figures envelopes me and I feel as though I'm sinking down into the mattress. I try to shout, but I cannot open my mouth. I panic when I suddenly realise I can't move a muscle in my body. I am totally paralysed. I try hard to fight back, but the most I can do is make a strange noise that comes from my throat. Hoping Margaret might hear me, I make another grunting sound, and my body feels like it's coming back to normal. The shadows have gone. As I look around the room, the nightlights give a warm welcoming glow, just enough to check on each corner of the room. I sing songs in my head to keep me awake, too frightened to fall asleep; however, I eventually drift into a peaceful sleep.

The next morning, in a tiny whisper of a voice, I tell Margaret about the shadows. A tear falls from my eye as I speak because it sounds so silly. Margaret makes me a cup of tea and sits beside me.

'I know you don't sleep properly anymore, I sometimes hear you in the night, in fact, once I heard you talking to someone and you scared the life out of me,' she laughs, 'I assumed you were talking in your sleep when it went quiet again, but to be on the safe side I did come down to check on you, and, if you remember, you were wide awake.'

I didn't remember, and Margaret continued.

'You've had a lot of dreams about shadows and dark hooded figures over the year's Dad. I wish there was something I could do to stop them. The dreams started when you began taking the medication for Parkinson's, or it could even be the disease itself, I don't know, but at least they're not as bad as they used to be.'

'They are.' I wanted to shout.

Margaret carried on talking. 'Only recently, I read an article about how people with Parkinson's only sleep an average of three hours before waking. I also found something interesting in a magazine last week, about people being unable to wake from a bad dream, similar to what you have. It's called Sleep Paralysis, and it's a lot more common than people think. Though it may seem to last a long time, it's only a few seconds or a couple of minutes, and usually happens when someone is just entering or leaving sleep. It's linked to REM, which indicates that someone is dreaming.'

I look at her in confusion.

'Rapid Eye Movement; you know Dad, you've seen it in babies when their eyelids are closed but their eyes are moving. That's what they call REM.'

I nod, but I'm not sure what she means really. We used to say it was wind that caused a baby's eyes to move when they were sleeping. I missed what Margaret was saying and she starts to explain again.

'When the body and brain enter REM sleep, the muscles relax and the brain blocks signals that would normally allow the limbs to move, so preventing the body from acting out its dreams. The article said it could be caused when sleeping and wakefulness temporarily co-inside, so some sleep phenomena, of which paralysis is one, breaks into wakefulness. In other words I suppose, it means the mind is awake but the body is asleep. Or is it the other way round?'

Jaysus, Mary and Joseph, now I really am confused.

'Oh and another thing' Margaret said just before leaving the room. 'As sleep paralysis causes anxiety, this can trigger a nightmare, but a waking nightmare. The article said that most people see shadows or a cloaked figure. It's funny when you think about it really. For centuries the black hooded figure has represented the Angel of Death . . . you know . . . the Grim Reaper, an image dressed in a dark cloak with a hood covering his face. But it was actually in the 15th century that the Grim Reaper took on this dark, hooded persona. Apparently, the image of a dark robed figure with a bowed head evolved from the traditional pallbearers at funerals. So I suppose you could say it's all in the mind . . . mmm,' she said, 'I wonder if the pressure in your chest is caused through fear. You know, being unable to breathe properly. Perhaps our fear of the Grim Reaper being a sign of death is just a figment of our imagination. It can't be real or we wouldn't all be here to tell the tale.'

She walked back to the bed and touched my hand.

'It's not a pleasant experience Dad, in fact it's an awful experience. I've had it myself a few times. It usually happens when I've been over tired. Unfortunately for you, it's much more common for people that sleep on their back.'

I can do little else then to sleep on my back.

Margaret walked into the kitchen and shouted back to me. 'Oh by the way, it has nothing to do with mental illness or anything like that, so don't be worrying about it.'

No, I won't worry. I'll just try to stay awake forever and ever, Amen, after hearing all that.

*

A lot has changed since coming out of hospital the last time. Because of the pressure sores on my heels, I'm unable to move around, or even stand on my feet at all. I'm all skin and bone now, so I suppose you could say I'm bed bound. My legs are twisted through locking together, and I have to sleep with a pillow between my knees. My body is giving up. I feel death really *is* all around me now and not in my imagination as I tried to convince myself. I see dead people, people from my past who have died; even my brother-in-law, Tom, who always shortened my name to Pat, came to see me last night.

'Hey up Pat,' he says, sitting on the edge of the bed, 'we're all waiting for you. You're dying, you know that don't you. You'll be OK Pat. We've been watching over you for a while now. All of us are here; ready to take care of you.'

'Tom.' I shouted, but he was gone in a second.

The following evening, I tried to tell Nicholas that Tom had been to see me, but all I could say was Tom. I couldn't get the words out. I heard him ask Margaret who Tom was and she explained to him it was Joyce's brother, and how very close we had been.

They say it's been six months since I have been bed bound, apart from going out twice. One was to go to Meadow Hall shopping centre, to get some new clothes for me, and the other time to visit the war museum, near York. Both trips caused a lot of problems, not only in getting me ready, but also because when we got there I was uncomfortable. It's very difficult to get me into my wheelchair from a hoist, and when I'm eventually sat in it, my trousers either slide down or ride up; and I lean to the left so they have to prop me up. I don't seem to have any strength left in my neck muscles, and holding my head up is extremely difficult. When we returned home, getting from the wheelchair back into bed was even more difficult, and we have all become reconciled, that it's best not to put me through the pain associated with transferring me from my bed, into the wheelchair, and visa versa.

I'm resigned to the fact that this is where I will have to stay from now on . . . in bed. I watch television, and can see people passing the house from the windows, and go through the years of my life to pass time on. My family come and visit, but I can no longer communicate with them, other than a few words. I remember when Patrick, my son, used to come down when Margaret and Geoff went out occasionally. We would watch Last of the Summer Wine and have a few lagers, and a laugh and a chat about the way we used to live in the fifties and sixties. I loved those nights and I miss them. Geoff would make us a supper before they set off, and once, Patrick took the folding tray from my lap to put it away.

'Let go Dad.' He said, pulling the tray away from me 'Dad let go of the tray.'

He pulled hard, taking my hand along with it. It took a while for him to realise my finger was stuck in the hinge, and I was trying to shout. When he did eventually realise what was happening, he said. 'You've got your finger stuck in the hinge.'

Taking a deep breath to enable me to get a sentence out, I shouted. 'Yeah that's what I was trying to tell you when you were dragging my finger off.'

We both laughed at the situation. He thought I was hanging onto to the tray, and I couldn't get the words out to tell him my finger was stuck.

Obviously, I realise that having Parkinson's disease has certainly changed my life. But to be honest, over the twelve years or so since being diagnosed, I've managed to live a normal life in most respects. In the last six years alone, from the age of seventy nine, I've travelled and seen a lot of places. Apart from the usual daytrips to the coast, the Yorkshire Dales, the Lake District and London; I have been to France, Ireland, and Wales and more recently, six months ago, I went on a visit to my grandson Adrian's house, in Devon. I'm grateful for the life I've had, and I suppose in some ways I have probably lived longer than I would have if I had been on my own. I was very depressed and unhappy after losing Joyce, and wonder how my life would have turned out if I had carried on drinking. I wasn't taking my medication on a regular basis when I was on my own, and I was drinking too much, so I suppose it's hard to say what would have happened.

My mind has been more alert than people have given me credit for, and if I could curse Parkinson's for anything, it would be for the loss of my voice. This was by far the hardest to bear. If it hadn't been for the recurrent water infections that were caused by both having to use a catheter and Parkinson's, then I would have had a better life still. The fact that a simple operation such as the Suprapubic catheter could have saved me all that misery and pain does make me angry; but the thing that upsets me most of all, is that these bed sores have stopped me in my tracks twice, and this time it's for good.

Parkinson's disease doesn't mean you have a death sentence, as I first thought, and there is no reason why someone with Parkinson's can't lead a reasonably normal life, once they have found the right medication. A lot of research has been going on throughout the years to find a cure, and I know it's too late for me, but hopefully in the not too distant future Parkinson's will, like many other diseases, be no longer heard of. Both Margaret and Geoff try to keep up to date on what's happening in the field of research for a cure, and sometimes tell me about the latest developments. Some experts believe the cause could lie within the environment and could be linked to pesticides building up in ground water. This is the water which lies just beneath the surface, and as all the chemicals farmers spray on the land seep through the soil, the water and the soil around it become saturated and toxic. For many years I worked digging and laying drainage pipes, not only on housing estates, but also on roads and motorways. I often came home from work covered in clay. For quite a few years I worked on the M62 motorway, that links Leeds and Manchester, as it runs through the countryside high up in the Pennines. Many were the days we were stood knee deep in stagnant water as we laid the long plastic tubes, which were to carry away the rain from the road surface. Three of my closest mates, who worked side by side with me, died from conditions that affected their memory and the balance of their minds, Dementia and Alzheimer's. Perhaps there is some truth in this theory. On the other hand, they do say depression can be the root cause of Parkinson's, and I have to admit when Joyce died I was very depressed, so maybe that was what started it.

I only ever had three wishes in my life where travel was concerned. One was to visit the war graves in Northern France; one was to see the Royal Edinburgh Military Tattoo in Scotland and lastly to go to the Vatican in Rome. I have fulfilled one wish, which was to see the war graves, and there was talk of going to Scotland this year to see the Tattoo, a wonderful sight that I watch every year on television. That would have fulfilled my second wish, but sadly I know it won't happen now. Although we often talked together about travelling to Rome, I knew in my heart travelling by plane was not an option, even some years ago. However, Margaret took me on a virtual tour of the Vatican using Google Earth, so you could say I got half my wish.

We have been through a lot, especially these past few years, but there have been some eventful times. I remember when Margaret's book was released and I was well and able enough to go to her book launch. It was good to meet up with family members I hadn't seen for years. The place was packed with people and she sold over one hundred copies in one night. The book continues to sell, and I got a lump in my throat when Geoff took me to see it sitting on the shelves of WHSmiths and Waterstones book shops. I remember too, a year later, when she was awarded a First Class Honours degree at the age of sixty two. I was honoured to sit in the front row for her big day when she graduated, and I clapped my hands together for everyone who received their scroll. Her final year dissertation was called 'Who Cares' and it was all about caring for someone with Parkinson's.

The night time shadows have long gone now. It's Joyce who comes to see me. I see her all the time, but I say nothing; although Margaret overheard me talking to her once through the baby alarm. She was surprised to hear me speak clearly for that very short time, just as I used to before I had Parkinson's. Joyce told me in a dream she would wait for me and she has kept that promise. The only woman I ever loved is waiting for me. Joyce takes away the fear of death, and perhaps that's why the night time shadows have stopped coming. I no longer fear them now. I see the sadness in my family's eyes when they look at me, and I know they hold back their tears for my sake. If I could speak, I would tell them I'm happy to go now. I would tell them the only regret is leaving my precious family behind, but I can't fight anymore. My story has to finish some time. It's 2012 and I am in my second millennium, my tenth decade and my eighty-fifth year. I've had a good run for my money and I am grateful for the time I spent with my lovely wife Joyce, and the life I have shared with our five children, my grandchildren and my great-grandchildren.

I'm back in hospital once more and I know I won't be home again. Not this time. I have my eyes closed most of the time but I am still aware. I'm aware that Geoff and my two daughters and three sons are with me urging me to get well. I hold on and try for their sakes, but I want to go now. Joyce is waiting and I'm too tired and exhausted to fight. I don't want to live as I have for the past months. I have spent the last six months in bed, being spoon fed and having my toilet needs seen to. Ironically, it's only eight months since Margaret and Geoff sent for a brochure to take me on a cruise, but the deterioration came quickly when I couldn't get out of bed, and I have wasted away. The muscles have ceased to work in my throat now and I can't speak at all. I can nod my head, but I can't shake it for no, only very slightly. After all this time, we have found other means of communicating, it's as if by intuition that Margaret knows exactly what I want to say. The doctors and nursing staff couldn't have tried any harder to make my last few days of life more comfortable. I have an air mattress and I am constantly being changed into different positions to help with the pressure sores. The sores may not be the reason I am dying, but they have given me the most discomfort; much more than Parkinson's ever did. Perhaps things are beginning to change now, and hopefully pressure sores will also be a thing of the past. I really hope so.

Life is never easy. Some of the hardest times give us our most profound memories and they make memories of happier times seem much more precious.

Appendix

It was 1817 when James Parkinson listed the main symptoms of a disease that now bears his name. His concerns about patients with tremors and a lack of ability to move freely, which he called 'Shaking Palsy' or 'Paralysis Agitans', have formed the basis on which Parkinson's disease is diagnosed today.

Almost two hundred years later, in 1998, the World Health Organisation stated that worldwide, there were approximately four million people who were affected by Parkinson's disease. Ten years later a report by Parkinson's UK, which is still considered relevant today, confirmed that every year throughout the United Kingdom there are approximately ten thousand individuals, one person every hour, who are diagnosed as having Parkinson's. This means that at any one time in the UK, about one hundred and twenty thousand people are trying to cope with the three major physical influences that are connected with this debilitating condition. The symptoms take the form of 'Tremor' where limbs or parts of the body may shake or make sudden uncontrollable movements, 'Rigidity' which often takes the form of stiffness in the joints, causing a reduction in supple movement and posture, and lastly 'Hypokinesis', an abnormal condition of diminished motor activity, which can result in a patient being unable to activate muscles or respond to signals from the brain.

Research has shown that Parkinson's is associated with a loss of dopamine producing nerve cells in the Substantia Nigra portion of the brain; which can cause other common symptoms such as stooping, shuffling, autonomic dysfunction and mental disorders, such as confusion and memory loss. The reason for these malfunctions is that Dopamine is a chemical that our brain uses to transmit signals to other parts of our brain, particularly areas that control motor function. As these brain cells die our ability to direct these signals diminishes and we start to lose control of parts of our body and mind. However the effects of Parkinson's disease are diverse and in general no two sufferers will be affected in the same way. This is because by the time of diagnosis, 60-80% of dopamine producing cells in the brain have died, and it is entirely dependent on which motor functions have been affected as to which symptoms will be prevalent. This means that the onset and prognosis of Parkinson's can be extremely varied and difficult to predict, and because the symptoms and progression of the disease are so unpredictable, a person may have the disease for years without knowing.

Most early symptoms of Parkinson's disease are generally mild and occur progressively. Many people may find these symptoms hard to explain, often keeping what is happening to them secret, hoping it is something that will pass. At first there may be just be a feeling of fatigue or a general sense of uneasiness, an awareness of a lack of energy, depression or trouble sleeping may be present and there may be a slight tremor or difficulty in standing. During the early stages about 70% of people experience a slight tremor in their hand or foot, and this is often restricted to one side of their body. Generally the tremor begins in the hands and arms and often involves the rubbing of the thumb against the forefinger and this becomes more obvious when the hand is at rest, or when they are under stress. As Parkinson's progresses, the tremors may affect other parts of the body as well, but not every person with Parkinson's has tremors. Although these tremors can be very distressing, they are usually not disabling and often disappear when you sleep.

As Parkinson's progresses, and it slowly begins to interrupt a person's daily activities, some people's speech becomes slurred, their handwriting changes, or the person may notice a stiffening or lack of movement. Often there is the absence of facial expressions and the muscles of the limbs and neck can become stiff and are unable to relax normally. Most develop some degree of rigidity, meaning that many may also experience aches, cramps or pains from these affected muscles, and occasionally the stiffness can be so severe that it limits movement altogether.

The disease usually gets worse over time and unfortunately to date there is no known cure. Although Parkinson's is not fatal; it is often other complications or illnesses which may occur and be exacerbated by Parkinson's, that lead to death.

*

It is not really known why Parkinson's disease develops in an individual. Some theories consider that chemicals found in standing water may be to blame, and indeed my father did come into contact with polluted water when he worked on the construction of the M62, as it was built across the Pennines. Others scientists are concerned that some individuals may be born with certain genes that may trigger Parkinson's and that isolating these genes may lead to earlier diagnosis or even lead to eventually finding a cure. However, an area that has been given great consideration, and one that I feel may easily have contributed to my father's disposition to Parkinson's, is that of stress and depression. It may have been a coincidence that my father's symptoms began to manifest themselves shortly after my mother died suddenly of cancer, but I am convinced that the process we all go through when faced with the difficulties of reacting to the death of a loved one, played a large part.

Previous generations were faced with a high percentage of deaths that affected babies, infants and young children. Indeed, the average life expectancy was much shorter than now, and so death was often considered a part of normal life. Whereas nowadays the most common causes of death are mostly the result of non-infectious chronic diseases, which tend to affect our ever growing elderly population, such as cancer, heart disease, diabetes, or respiratory failure; and often there is little or no warning to prepare us.

As with death, the role of grief in our lives has changed. It could be argued that when death strikes early or is a more regular event, our period of grief must, by association, be tempered and shortened. On the other hand, when grief comes later in life and strong bonds have been built, grief may perhaps be amplified and be much more long lasting. Initially there is often shock, even

214

when the death may have been expected, and this can be portrayed as disbelief or guilt, often manifesting itself as anger in both thought and deed. These phases of grief are not the same for each individual and can occur, or even be absent, yet sometimes reappear without warning. Frequently these initial feelings can be quickly replaced by anxiety. Not only with regard to what may happen in the future, about arrangements and financial considerations etc, but also how the way the deceased was treated when they were alive, is perceived. Did we do everything we could for them . . . could we have done more?

When faced with single traumatic events, such as the loss of a spouse, or partner, the person left behind will often suffer from reactive depression. As the phrase suggests, the individual will react to this event which has confronted them by feeling guilty. They may make unrealistic self evaluations and become predisposed with grief. The results of these feelings are that the person will often report a reduced ability to concentrate, become easily distracted, or be unable to make decisions. As a method of escaping from the realities that face them, they may have difficulty in remembering things and may become preoccupied with past failings. Frequently, thoughts of death or even suicide can manifest themselves. Fortunately, instances of suicide are infrequent, as it is a presumption of human existence to try and make the most of things, and this usually leads to a resumption, if somewhat slowly, of a more proactive approach to carrying on.

It isn't easy for anyone to come to terms with losing someone they love; but in my father's case, and for many more men of his era, suddenly taking on the responsibility of cooking, shopping, and doing household chores, came as a shock. In their generation, a married couple each had a role to play. Traditionally men went out to work and carried out repairs in the home and garden, whereas women stayed at home, raising children, cooking and cleaning. It was very rare to see a man hanging washing out on the line, cleaning windows, or standing over a stove. On the other hand, once the first child had been born the average women didn't get the chance to go out to work. Of course, this is not true of everyone, but for most families, that was how it was. Even after retirement, my father didn't shop, unless he went with my mother, he didn't cook or use the washing machine, tumble dryer and so on. Not because he wouldn't, but because my mother had played that role from first marrying him, and she continued to do so. She looked after him. Sadly, without her, my father found this new way of life hard, even with the help he received from his family. He'd not only lost his wife, but his friend and adviser, and it wasn't long before he became very depressed.

Whatever it was that initially triggered Parkinson's in my father; it was at this point in time that he needed the services and guidance of his local general practitioner. Normally, General Practitioners are our first port of call when we are faced with a serious illness. Psychologists often refer to them as the 'Gate Keepers' of the vast and confusing resource, which, in the United Kingdom, is the National Health Service. The term, gate keeper, is extremely apt as they hold the key to the initial evaluation, diagnosis and treatment which each patient's symptoms will require. Our GPs are also the cornerstone of the medical profession, as initially, many patients don't need a barrage of costly laboratory or clinical tests, nor do they need immediate specialist intervention. What is required, when doctors make a diagnosis or pass on information to a patient, is good communication. This is central to good medicine and needs to be a process of joint interaction between doctor and patient when transferring information as this reduces unnecessary uncertainty in either party. The patient should do their best to give a full account of their symptoms, and the doctor should respond by listening to, empathising with and reassuring the patient. In most cases this will produce sufficient information for the GP to make a full diagnosis, and improve the perception of a healthy prognosis and the prevention of unhealthy attitudes and outcomes. After all, the patient has attended the surgery to search for an expert's knowledge, and to couple that knowledge with any treatment that may be required.

At this point it is important to clarify that in some circumstances, patients are not comfortable with honest attempts to inform them of certain aspects of their illness, required treatment or prognosis. Often a patient, who feels they are seriously ill, can become dependent on the authoritative figure of a medical practitioner; preferring the doctor to take the responsibility of providing a solution. In recent times it has become the 'norm' for the medical profession to explain in great detail, the risks involved in procedures and prognosis, before placing the onus on the patient. Perhaps this may not always be desirable.

The onset of an illness often means that everyday routines are disrupted, and the sufferer is likely to feel both mentally and physically unwell for a period of time. Often this experience will be short lived, as with the common cold, for example, but in the case of a chronic illness such as Parkinson's disease, the impact on the sufferer's life and those around them will inevitably be more profound. If we cannot rely on our bodies and minds to function normally, then our self-esteem and possibly our interaction with others may become strained, and our dependency on close family members and friends may make an already problematic situation worse. To combat these feelings of uncertainty and inadequacy, individuals need an explanation not only of their symptoms, but also clear information on what the future may hold for them.

The pressure placed upon modern doctor patient relationships, and the time allotted for medical consultation, dictate that many patients may leave a consultation with little or no information. In most cases there is no longer the time for a "good bedside manner" where a GP or consultant can take the time to explain in great detail the ramifications of a patient's condition. To add to this problem many patients are reluctant to discuss their individual needs because they feel that it is unacceptable to do so, and may lead to them being judged as inadequate.

Though there are some areas of the country where specialist nurses are available, this availability can often fluctuate considerably, and whether or not a patient can access their services will depend largely on the NHS postcode lottery of catchment areas. Financial and physical considerations, imposed by successive governments, have transferred the necessity of learning about an illness onto the patient, and not all patients have the inclination or capacity to access this information. Patients feel out of their depth, are in denial, or simply do not know where to look.

Though there are organisations that can offer an in-depth and comprehensive insight into chronic illness, not everyone is predisposed to joining a formal organisation or group. An individual's tendency to search for, and source information, will therefore depend on the ease in which this information is made available.

In recent years, it has been suggested that the use of a computer with internet access has opened up a new vista for information and education retrieval, and it cannot be denied that there is indeed a wealth of knowledge at our fingertips. There are however, concerns as to how those sections of society, especially older members who have not grown up with computer technology, or indeed may not readily have access to a computer, will be able to gain this knowledge. A combination of these factors could mean the patients knowledge of their symptoms, or treatment and the prognosis of their illness will remain deficient.

In order for people who suffer from chronic illnesses to live safer and more fulfilled lives, it is of paramount importance that the Medical Profession, as a whole, but particularly health psychologists, health information promoters and charitable organisations, should be able to provide adequate, coherent information regarding the nature of the affliction, and the most effective means of coping with and self-regulating the condition. It is also imperative that the patient, or end user, should be made fully aware of the existence of this invaluable source of knowledge.

It is gratifying to know that over the past two decades, most GPs understand these issues, and are now extremely competent in making sure that their patients have belief, not only in the changes that could be used to combat, or alleviate their illness or disease, but also in their own ability to be able to make these changes.

*

In general, there is a time delay between being diagnosed and the onset of any real need for formal caring. This is because Parkinson's disease is a slowly progressing disorder and it is quite common for many patients to go a number of years before significant changes in their initial symptoms appear. When patients continue to be physically and mentally fit, and have a full and rewarding lifestyle, both at home and often in their business environment, many of them can become content with their situation, and continue to make the most of their lifestyle.

One such person was Janet Reno, who in 1995 was the United States Attorney General, during President Clinton's term of office. It was during a brisk morning walk, surrounded by FBI agents, that she first noticed a slight tremor in her left hand. She went to see her doctor, who confirmed the presence of Parkinson's disease, suggesting that she would probably be fine for twenty years. When asked if he thought Parkinson's would affect her ability to serve as attorney general, he confirmed that she should use her time well. For many years Janet Reno continued her political life as she remained the attorney general, and even ran, all be it unsuccessfully, for the governorship of the state of Florida.

These experiences, where there are no major symptom difficulties, are common among early stage sufferers of the disease. Many will lead full and active lives, socialising with friends and family and taking regular holidays. However, the implications of Parkinson's disease cannot be overestimated and it is important that individuals be prepared for their future circumstances. Not only by understanding the consequences of Parkinson's disease, but also by being mentally prepared for the stresses which are likely to occur, once the condition progresses and care is needed.

The periods just before and immediately after being diagnosed had to be the worst time for my father. He was confused and frightened. We were at a loss as to know what to do for him, and I suppose we put things down to the side effects of his new medication; after all, this is when he seemed to have changed. He slept throughout the day, which was not only bad for his posture, but also very confusing because of all the dreams he was having. He had no life as such, as he had previously. I felt at this point we were losing my father. He seemed to have lost the will to live. He was tired and weary and the hallucinations brought him terrible misery.

It is not the intention of this book to try to explain the complicated and intricate array of Parkinson's drugs, or the technical medical way in which they work. This, quite rightly, needs to be left to the medical experts who have written many interesting and informative books on the subject, and for the individual reader to decide if they wish to pursue this avenue of research.

What has most definitely been recognised, and was very apparent during the years of caring for my father, is that people who are afflicted with Parkinson's need their medication at regular intervals. Once again, each individual need will be different. The balance of how much medication, and how often it is taken, may take many weeks and months to work out, and often this is the result of a great deal of trial and error. However once a regime has been found to work, it is vital that the individual's medication is administered at the required times throughout the day or night. Deviation from these times, even by so much as an hour, can cause problems as the balance of their body chemicals can be severely disrupted. This can lead to a noticeable negative difference in the person taking the medication. Excessive disruption to this strict regime, by completely missing as little as one dose of the prescribed amount of medication, could result in an uneven release of Dopamine, which can have a problematic effect on digestion, sleep patterns and bodily functions.

During the years of caring for my father, there were many instances when his medication was delayed and even missed. On each and every occasion it was found that the problems created could take hours, days or weeks to stabilise, before allowing him to return to his "normal" life.

When determining and administering the form of treatment and medication that a patient may receive, the medical profession can often bring about a situation where non medical intervention is frowned upon, and often discouraged. In the case of family members and carers, many health professionals are guilty of not recognising the importance of their input into decision making. They often think of them as 'next of kin' rather than considering them as a valuable source of background information and a deep well of knowledge about the patient. After all, these individuals often spend twenty four hours a day, usually seven days a week, being party to all the symptoms and difficulties that the patient faces, and as the decisions the medical professionals are making, can often be life changing decisions and judgments; excluding relatives and carers can produce a dual dilemma. In the first place, many family members and carers will have to face making judgments about the correctness and value of their own actions. Should they act to initiate or prevent something from happening, especially when the result could be life threatening? And secondly, should they, for the patient's welfare, take the risk of alienating the medical staff?

The ultimate implementation and acceptance of these actions will depend on the carer's own personal code of ethics, and may often culminate in making some people afraid or anxious. Perhaps a much more cooperative outcome in the case of close family and medical interaction would be if both parties could offer recognition, information and support without feeling under any kind of threat.

Take the case of my experience as a close relative, and as a carer. I have often been faced with situations where I have felt pushed out and been ignored. There have been many occasions where, due to the lack of specialist knowledge about Parkinson's disease, members of the medical staff have not been fully understanding about the needs of my father's condition. These needs can manifest themselves as a minor consideration, such as the simple need for extra pillows to support his head, or be more harmful, and be both physically and psychologically damaging; such as when his medication was administered at the hospitals convenience, rather than his normal routine. Medical staff must address the important fundamental principle, that because Parkinson's disease carries such a wide range of underlying symptoms, it can be very easy for individual patients to be completely misunderstood. Many people who have Parkinson's can seem to be perfectly normal, whatever normal may be, and outwardly their Parkinson's symptoms can mask their underlying difficulties. In the case of my father, apart from his tremor, which was significantly controlled by medication, and the stiffness in his neck joints, at this time, he did not really show much in the way of symptoms. Unfortunately for him, one of the unseen problems caused by his condition was that his short term memory was affected, and he was finding it difficult, not only to remember things and events that had happened recently, but also to draw a parallel between these events and questions he was expected to answer. There were to be many instances when people made the false assumption, that because his mind was not able to answer questions quickly enough, he must be either deaf or suffering from dementia. I am glad to say that on many occasions my father would be the first to dismiss this misconception.

The district nurses were always very good to my father, and talked through each stage of the treatment he was being given. They had respect for him and for us also, as we cared for him, as did the doctors who came to visit him over the years. But I do believe the people who run our hospitals need to reassess their priorities, and the same goes for the medical teams in hospitals, concerning the way they approach patient care; especially when the patient is cared for by a spouse or close relatives. It was difficult for my father, as he couldn't speak for himself, or remember his recent symptoms, relying on one of us to answer for him.

When medics gather around a patients bed to assess them, or to do simple tasks, such as putting on their pyjamas, or taking blood; they always ask the family members to wait outside. In some cases, when the visitors are not close family members, this may be necessary, but I am sure that relatives, who are often the main carers, know more about the patient's condition than the patients do themselves. They often spend twenty four hours a day coping with all the ailments and difficulties of dealing with their loved ones condition. Surely their expertise and knowledge could be invaluable to a hospital staff that is, in the main, dedicated to making their patients well again. Perhaps a bringing together of the skills of both the medical profession, and the often untrained, but effective skills of the carer, would put an end to people suffering avoidable distress, such as being bed bound with pressure sores. Three days is a long time for someone to be in the same position.

Seventy two hours of not being moved; simply because the nurses don't have the time.

The use of alternative therapies to help combat the symptoms of Parkinson's is not as common as perhaps it might be. Conceivably, this is because Parkinson's disease is not widely understood by alternative therapy practitioners, or perhaps it is because people who have Parkinson's are baffled by the numerous types of therapies that are advertised, particularly on the internet.

In my opinion, there are aspects of Parkinson's disease where clinical hypnosis may help a person to alleviate some of the day to day symptoms, such as releasing stress and helping with depression. It may also be possible to help reduce tremor and shaking by the use of triggers that will help a person relax their muscles, and though I would never claim that hypnosis could totally alleviate these symptoms, it should not be discounted. Hypnosis brings about a state of total relaxation where the mind can be open to beneficial suggestions and, should nothing come from this, the person who is undergoing hypnosis will awaken completely relaxed.

There are of course, many other forms of alternative therapy which could have a beneficial effect, and perhaps the most obvious of these would be Massage. This is often the simplest and most effective method of relieving tension and stiffness in people with Parkinson's, and when coupled with the use of the Alexander Technique, may combat leaning and poor posture. Other therapies that are relatively easy to access are, Yoga, which has been used in India to promote good balance, posture and flexibility for over five thousand years, and from China, Tai Chi, which teaches co-ordination of the mind and breathing, whilst helping with balance and posture. Both of these therapies have exercises which can be performed in a sitting position, which may be of assistance to Parkinson's patients.

In recent years there has been some credibility given to therapies that may not be immediately apparent, and yet, once suggested, their benefits are obvious. Therapies such as Singing, which helps considerably with throat muscles and breathing, Dance, which again aids posture and general fitness, and Art and Pet therapies which both promote wellbeing. All of these and many more alternative therapies should not be discounted, as anything that is carried out sensibly and can work alongside Parkinson's traditional medication, must be of benefit.

I am convinced the sessions of guided imagery which my father took part in, went a long way to helping him re-establish his determination to walk again, and lead as normal a life as he could. The ordeal he had suffered because of the treatment he had received in hospital, the subsequent pressure sores, and the long rehabilitation period he needed, took an enormous amount out of him. Indeed, if he had only had to contend with his Parkinson's symptoms, he would probably not have been greatly inconvenienced. He was of course still in the mid stages of the disease, and it is perfectly possible he may have only had to endure the normal conditions associated with gradually growing old gracefully. I have to say, I admired his determination as he spent the summer and autumn regaining his strength, and learning how to walk. He would walk up and down the garden using his three wheeled walking aid, day after day, until he was able to use his walking stick as before.

He did start to walk our dog around the playing field again, though it took a few months before we could bring ourselves to let him go on his own, and even then I could not resist keeping an eye on him. His gait was much slower now and I suppose it was just as well that Bonnie was slowing down too. It was really heart-warming to see them both strolling along, stopping to meet up with old friends, both human and canine, and they managed to continue until the winter weather made walking impossible. Of course he finally accepted that if we were going somewhere which involved a lot of walking, he would need to use his wheelchair, but as much as possible he would manage by just using his stick.

*

The fluctuating symptoms which are associated with Parkinson's disease, can often result in a tremendous strain on the lives, not only of the person with Parkinson's, but also on the physical and mental health of the spouse or carer. Indeed, in a large percentage of carer patient relationships, involving people with Parkinson's, the spouse often takes on the role of principle carer. In many cases, this can bring about a rise in the levels of stress and emotional pressures that are associated with, not only coming to terms with their partner's condition, but also being able to cope with the emotional and physical factors, which will present themselves whilst carrying out the role of the carer.

When a patient is discharged from hospital there is often an assessment of the needs of the patient, when every attempt is made to determine their daily needs. This can take the form of pre-discharge house visits or simply clarification that the patients needs can be met. In general, little is done to assess, or address, the implications of the discharge on close relatives or carers. Often, the only contact a spousal carer will have with primary healthcare professionals will be during visits from district nurses, or occupational therapists. In either case, the emphasis on any intervention will generally focus on the patient, rather than the carer.

One of the greatest burdens placed upon carers of people with Parkinson's disease is that of falling. The prospect of always having to be on the lookout for potential falls. Involuntary movements, loss of balance and stiffness which can increase the possibility of falling, can often lead the carer to become agitated and resentful of the burden that has been placed upon them. A secondary, and yet often a more devastating consequence of a fall, can be when the carer or spouse injure themselves carrying out whatever method they employ in trying to raise the fallen person off the ground. This can be extremely dangerous and traumatic, particularly when the person who has fallen is incapable of providing any form of assistance, thereby becoming a dead weight, and making the task almost impossible. Unfortunately, one of the recourses taken by many carers can be to restrict the amount of movement enjoyed by the person they are caring for. It can be extremely demanding when the carer has to spend enormous amounts of time watching for potential falls, or other dangerous occurrences, and this can significantly limit the quality of life for both parties.

In the case of my father, and his propensity to fall, the majority of these occasions were thankfully limited to when he was feeling strong enough to move around under his own steam. It was not often that he would just stand up and collapse to the ground; it was more that he would be on the move when, for a variety of reasons, he would slide or slump to the floor. Sometimes, one leg would involuntarily move across the other and he would trip, and then again, sometimes it would be a shear loss of balance that would cause him to fall. He was, however, determined not to let these falls deter him from moving around, and I am quite convinced it was his determination to keep mobile which promoted the suppleness in his body, and his perception of when falls were likely to happen.

Having someone else to help in the event of a fall cannot be over emphasised, and because Geoff and I were usually on hand together, we could manage most situations. I cannot imagine how difficult it must be for a spousal carer to have to be able to manage on their own, and I can only have empathy and understanding for people who are faced with the dilemma of falling. Sadly, many spouses are faced with an unassailable task, and due to practical or emotional reasons, the problem of falling often forces many spouses to reluctantly resort to placing their loved ones into a home.

*

It was heart breaking to see the dramatic change in my father when the pressure sores on his heels forced him to stay in bed. As the weeks wore on, I knew he had given up the fight and would fight no more. It was a struggle to persuade him to eat, and without disrespect to my father, it was like trying to feed a baby. His head would turn away from the spoon, and we had to constantly coax him to eat the smallest amount of food. We knew it was because he was losing his independence, and the ability to feed himself. I think we could probably have overcome the difficulties of getting him to eat if it had not been for the demeaning daily necessity of attending

226

to his toiletry needs. The acute pain in his heels meant he could no longer stand, even holding onto his frame, and I saw the look in his eyes as he was washed and dressed each day, whilst he lay on the bed. The only way he could be moved was to use the hoist to lift and lower him onto a wheeled commode chair, and then with the aid of a special ramp that Geoff had built, he could be taken to be showered and do the other necessities. I knew my father recognised the inevitability of his circumstances and considered them undignified, and I often wonder at this stage would a person die out of choice, if given the chance.

I have nothing but admiration for my husband Geoff. On each of the designated days, he would be on hand when the nurse came to change my father's dressings, and on the other days he would see to the wounds himself, carefully cleaning the sores and renewing the dressings. The smell from the pressure sores was horrendous, and when the dressings were being changed, the whole house was filled with the odour. Both Geoff and I were extremely grateful for the essential dedication that was shown by the district nurses, as over the weeks and months the treatment of my father's sores began to show improvement. Gradually, even though he still could not put his weight on them, the deep wounds began to fill with new flesh, and the skin reformed until the only sign was a small dent in his heel, surrounded by bright pink skin.

Even at this stage of his illness, my father didn't like me being in the room when he was getting dressed, and this put a huge responsibility on Geoff's shoulders. On one occasion, my father had slipped down the side of the bed while Geoff was trying to change his pyjamas, and was stuck. He had to lift him back onto the bed on his own, and I was relieved that Geoff didn't end up hurting himself. There was also a time, when I was in hospital myself. Geoff had taken my father to the bathroom, and was in the process of transferring him back to his wheelchair before hoisting him back into bed, when my father collapsed. Geoff could barely hold him up and there was no one else in the house. Fortunately, he managed to stretch out, still holding my father, and reach the telephone, which was just outside the shower room door on the desk. He called for an ambulance, explaining to the lady on the telephone what the situation was. She realised the urgency and arranged for the ambulance to come immediately. The ambulance crew took my father's weight off Geoff and helped to lift him back into bed.

As with the doctors and district nurses, the ambulance service has also been second to none over the years. On more than one occasion they had to be called out when I was on my own, to help lift my father and check him over for injuries. On each of the times, whether to take my father into hospital, or just to check him over, they were always so very pleasant, laughing and joking with him. After all, the entire situation of Geoff struggling to hold on to my father, to prevent him banging his head on the tiles, could have developed into something much more serious, and their services would most definitely have been needed.

Time again, we were told by other people that my father should be in a home. To us, he was in a home . . . his own home, a home where he had carers who cared. We couldn't give in now; we had come so far, although I have nothing but sympathy and respect for people that do have to resort to putting a loved one into care. It must be extremely difficult for some people to carry on caring for their loved ones, especially when they are on their own.

My father was literally, all skin and bone towards the end. There was very little flesh on his body, and his eyes seemed to grow large, with an almost frightened gaze to them. He had no appetite and was reluctant to drink water, and sometimes it hurt me, thinking I was being cruel, as I begged him to eat a little and drink fluids. The only food he was happy to eat was rice pudding or custard, and I realise the reason was because it was easy to swallow. For years he had bounced back from infections associated with Parkinson's, but the disease didn't stop him living a good life; it was the pressure sores that not only accelerated his decline, but also took away his spirit.

*

Who then, is to look after the thousands of people with Parkinson's disease and cater for their needs? As the majority of Parkinson's sufferers are over fifty years of age, most of that care will probably be provided by relatives, who in most cases will be their spouse/partner. The needs of Parkinson's carers are a very important component of the long term care of Parkinson's patients. This is because caring for people with Parkinson's in their own homes by close relatives, spouses or partners, is an important reason why many Parkinson's patients are institutionalised much later than those who are cared for by more professional caring bodies. The reason for this is that many family members, who provide care, will only succumb to long term institutionalisation when their own inability to cope is reached; and this is often when they are consumed by physical or emotional pressures.

It is the nature of Parkinson's disease, and its frequent symptoms, of both physical and mental impairment and depression, which can have a huge impact on the lives of both the patient and the carer; and it is vital that we understand the problems faced by carer/spouses. Surveys of Parkinson's caregivers have shown that there are many aspects of care-giving that will raise concerns for care-givers, reporting many problem areas, such as physical tiredness, being physically ill, marriage deterioration, loss of their social life and depression. Caregiver distress is often linked to Parkinson's disease severity, though strangely enough mental symptoms, such as dementia and cognitive impairment, are often considered less stressful than motor impairment. This could possibly be that difficulties in movement, and a greater likelihood of falls, are considered more likely to produce problems. However, bouts of depression in the patient will be the strongest influence on carer distress, often leading to carer depression. Depression in a patient is therefore a strong predictor of carer depression, poor psychological health and a decline in mental status.

It is mainly spousal caregivers who are subjected to these physical and emotional pressures. This can cause stress to build up and often results in sadness and the onset of depression. When compared with non-caring healthy elderly people, carers of people with Parkinson's are much more likely to suffer long standing illness or disability than non carers, and often the strain on wives' morale is significantly more than that of husbands'. Carers can often neglect their own well being as their experience of caring becomes more intense, and carers must not be allowed to become overwhelmed by what is required; nor should carers reach a stage where they are physically exhausted. Caring is an interpersonal process based on the characteristics of both the carer and the care recipient and sometimes there can be a breakdown in the relationship between carer and those being cared for and even elder abuse can occur. Quality of life can deteriorate, and the needs of carers and patients will be widespread. These areas may easily include mobility, carer relief, respite, financial support, spiritual needs and the need for professional services.

One of the major reasons why many carers can be traumatised by the fear of medical, and social service intervention, is the threat of their loved ones being taken away from them. This will often be the reason why carers, particularly spouses, will not ask for help, and will sometimes hide the difficulties they are experiencing, being reluctant to discuss their individual needs with health professionals. Perhaps the reason people suffer in silence is they feel society considers it is unacceptable to admit there are problems, and may lead to them being judged as inadequate. Should this situation arise, well co-ordinated and integrated assistance needs to be readily available. Most carers feel they are supported by their GPs, but find that district nurses are too busy to be proactive in helping carers, and some medical services and social services need to be more easily contactable.

Surveys have found that often the most psychologically demanding experiences for a carer/spouse can be when they feel they have lost contact with old friends and family. This can cause feelings of isolation, and isolation does not have to be outside the family home, many carer/spouses can feel isolated inside the home itself. Caring for a relative with a chronic and debilitating disease has far reaching implications for a carer's social activities. Carer/spouses are less likely to leave the house, have regular holidays, or to continue contact with friends and neighbours, particularly during the advanced stages of Parkinson's disease. However, many carers/spouses are less bothered by social dysfunction, but are more concerned about their fears and emotional functioning, and their ability to cope with their physical capabilities. Bonding with their partners, families or friends was seen as being the least of their problems. A family's financial, physical and emotional resources can test a families best coping skills, and family members, who are not regularly associated with the daily care of people with Parkinson's disease, often find the task daunting. This can often result in an increase in the time spent away from the family environment, and a lapse in communication between sections of the extended family. Having lost contact with many of their friends and some of their family, this lack of family support can be a major reason for full time nursing home care being contemplated.

Over one third of older people can expect to care for someone in retirement, and a predominant reason for spouses to relinquish the responsibility of care and the subsequent provision of care home facilities, is the ill health of the carer/spouse. Many people feel unable to continue caring for their loved one because coping with the needs of a spouse, particularly one who is in the later stages of Parkinson's, can involve caring duties that will tax even the most dedicated of individuals. This can sometimes leave them feeling overwhelmed and physically depleted. Finding the right care home and deciding to make use of these facilities is not a decision to be taken lightly, as there will be concerns and worries about some aspects of the care. Difficulties can arise from a lack of privacy and carers/spouses, who want to continue helping their partners, are often discouraged by the staff of care homes. This can result in the disempowerment and alienation of the caregiver and some carer/spouses report that their relationship with their partners deteriorated, even though they made frequent or even daily visits to the home.

Hopefully the role played by carers of Parkinson's disease sufferers will gradually becoming more recognised, and a carer's confidence in their ability and decisions, will grow with experience. There are care-givers who recognise benefits arising from being a carer. One of the most poignant articles I have ever read, concerning the intensity of caring for someone with Parkinson's disease, was written in The Times newspaper on Sept 21st 2009. In this article Judith Magill recounts how her husband was diagnosed with Parkinson's disease, and how for four years little altered. Then progressively he began to find normal everyday events difficult. There were also deeper changes too: eating, drinking, washing and dressing became a major effort. Judith explained that she had to do everything for him, including his toilet. He became a twenty four hour responsibility, and she felt that her husband's role had changed into that of a patient. Judith makes a very important observation when she reports: the world of the disabled is not only small, it is full of potential humiliation, and yet, she states, there are compensations. There can be a stronger bond, and sharing everyday chores can produce an intimacy that is intense and relationships can grow stronger. In her own words she explains:

"When your husband tells you he cannot live without you, it is normally a romantic exaggeration: with us, it is the literal truth"

The United Kingdom and much of the western world is facing a paradigm shift in healthcare provision, when major changes must take place to cater for the new burden that our growing elderly population will place upon both health and social care. Primary health care and social services have already been required to work more closely together, because of the failure of the two services to meet the needs of integrated care; and there is still a huge chasm between the amount of help that is available for carers, and the potential benefits of resourceful caring that is untapped in families, especially in the case of spouses. The ways that professional services, across a broad spectrum of health and social care, could be redirected and mobilised to make sure that carer/spouses are in a position to give Parkinson's sufferers adequate care at home, is limitless. Effective home care would relieve pressure on providing specialised institutionalised care homes, both financially, through the huge savings on building costs and interest repayments, and in terms of human resources in the recruitment and training of professional caring and nursing staff. However, should institutional care become unavoidable, every effort should be made to make it environmentally friendly for both patient and spouse, and the involvement of spousal input into the daily care regime must be paramount. Inclusion of carer's views on their potential role in care involvement, and the alleviation of stigma and the stresses associated with placing a spouse into care must be reconciled.

In conclusion; as the eventual requisites of caring for the needs of people with Parkinson's is so diverse, healthcare professionals, social agencies, charitable organisations, and present and prospective carer/spouses of people with Parkinson's disease may hold the key to unlocking this paradigm shift in care implementation; and this diversity could help many other individuals, whatever their ailment or condition might be.

Bibliography

Aarsland, D., Larsen, J.P., Karlsen, K., Lim, N.G. and Tanberg, E. (1999) Mental symptoms in Parkinson's disease are important contributors to caregiver distress *International Journal of Geriatric Psychiatry* 14, 866-874(1999)

Armitage, G., Adams, J., Newell, R., Coates, D., Ziegler, L. and Hodgson, I. (2009) Caring for persons with Parkinson's disease in care homes: Perceptions of residents and their close relatives, and an associated review of residents' care plans *Journal of Research in Nursing* 2009 14: 333 [on-line] Available from http://jm.sagepub.com/content/14/4/333 [Date accessed] 6 November 2010

Bridges-web, C., Giles, B., Speechly,C., Zurynski, Y. and Hiramanck, N. (2006) Patients with dementia and their cares in general practice *Australian Family Physician*: Volume 25 No. 11 November 2006. [on-line] Available at; http://www.racgp.org.au/afp/200611/20061103webb.pdf [Accessed 29 December 2010]

Brown, B. B. (1984) *Between health and Illness*: Houghton Mifflin

Brunt, M. (1982) Physiology *in Nursing*: Harper & Row.

Bumagin, V. and Hirn, K. (2006) Care-giving: A guide to those who give care and those who receive it: Springer Publishing [on-line] Available at http://site.ebrary.com/lib/uoh/doc [accessed] 25 January 2010

Caird, F. J. (1999) The importance of psychological symptoms in Parkinson's disease: *Age and Aging* 1999; 28; 335-336 [on-line]

Calder, S. A., Ebmeler, K.P., Stewart, L.,Crawford, J.R. and Besson, J.A.O.(1991) The prediction of stress in carers: The role of behaviour, reported self care and dementia in patients with idiopathic Parkinson's disease *International Journal of Geriatric Psychiatry* Volume 6, Issue 10, October 1999, pp 737-742

Cheung, J. and Hocking, P. (2004) Caring as worrying: the experience of spousal carers In *The Journal of Advanced Nursing* 47(5), 475-482
http://onlinelibrary.wiley.com.librouter.hud.ac.uk/doi/10.1111/j.13
65-2648.2004.03126.x/pdf

Cifu, D.X., Carne, W., Brown, R., Pegg, P., Ong, J., Qutubuddin, A. and Baron, M.S. (2006) Caregiver distress in Parkinsonism *Journal of Rehabilitation Research & Development* Volume 43, November 4, pp 499-508

Clarke, C. E., Gullaksen, E., Macdonald, S. and Lowe, F. (1999) Referral criteria for speech and language therapy assessment of swallowing caused by idiopathic Parkinson's disease In Percival, R. and Hobson, P. Eds. *Parkinson's Disease: Studies in Psychological and Social Care*: BPS Books. PP246-255

Collins, C. and Jones, R. (1997) Emotional distress and morbidity in dementia carers: a matched comparison of husbands and wives. *International Journal of Geriatric Psychiatry*: Volume 12: 1168-1173 (1997) {on-line]

Cousins, R., Davies, A., Playfer, J. and Turnbull, C. (1999) *Caring for the carers*: [on-line] Available from:
http://radcliffepublishing.com/books/samplechapters/1149

D'Amelio, M., Terruso, V., Palmeri, B., Benedetto, N.D., Famoso, G., Cottone, P., Aridon, P., Ragonese, P. And Savettieri, G. (2009) Predictors of caregiver burden in patients with Parkinson's disease *Neurol Sci* (2009) 30:171-174 [on- line] Available from: http://www.springerlink.com/content/a7895l33355132v1/ [Accessed 26 October 2010]

Davey, C., Wiles, R., Ashburn, A. and Murphy, C. (2004) Falling in Parkinson's disease: the impact on informal caregivers *Disability and Rehabilitation* 2004, Vol. 26, No 23, Pages 1360-1366.

Davies, A.D.M., Cousins, R., Turnbull, C. J., Playfer, J. R. and Bromley, D. B. (1999) The experience of caring for people with Parkinson's disease In Percival, R. and Hobson, P. Eds. *Parkinson's Disease: Studies in Psychological and Social Care*: BPS Books. PP154-198

Elias, J. W. and Hutton, T. (1999) Causes and Prevention of Falls in Parkinson's Disease In Hutton, T. J. and Dippel, R. L. (1999) *Caring for the Parkinson's Patient*: Eds. Prometheus Books

Foster. M. A. (2011) Who Cares. A degree dissertation held at Huddersfield University.

Happe, S. and Berger, K. (2002) The association between caregiver burden and sleep disturbances in partners and patients with Parkinson's disease. In *Oxford Journal of Age and Aging:* Volume 31, Issue 5, p 349-354 [on-line].

Hobson, P., Leeds, L. and Meara, J. (2001) The coping methods of patients with Parkinson's disease, their carers, and the associations between health-related quality of life and depression *Quality in Aging and Older Adults* Volume 2 Number 4/ December 2001 [On-line] Available at
http://pierprofessional.metapress.com/content0616075xp7684g13/

[Accessed 6 November 2010]

Hutton, J.T. and Dippel, R.L. (1999) *Caring for the Parkinson Patient*: Prometheus Books

Jones, R., D'eath, C., Harnsford, J., Hutchinson, H., Hyde, L., Thurlow, L. A and Spanton, L. (1999) The needs of people with Parkinson's disease and their families: the Parkinson's disease study, Devon and Cornwall, 1989-92 In Percival, R. and Hobson,

P. Eds. *Parkinson's Disease: Studies in Psychological and Social Care*: BPS Books. PP60-78

Lesser, R. and Whitworth, A. (1999) Communication in Parkinson's disease with cognitive impairment: a diagnostic and therapeutic medium? In Percival, R. and Hobson, P. Eds. *Parkinson's Disease: Studies in Psychological and Social Care*: BPS Books. PP236-245

Lieberman, A.N. and Williams, F. (1995) *Parkinson's disease The Complete Guide for Patients and Carers*: Thorsons.

Lloyd, M. (1999) The new community care for people with Parkinson's disease and their carers In Percival, R. and Hobson, P. Eds. *Parkinson's Disease: Studies in Psychological and Social Care*: BPS Books. PP 13-59

Lloyd, M. (2000) Where has All the Care Management Gone? The Challenge of Parkinson's Disease to the Health and Social Care Interface *British Journal of Social Work* (2000) 30, 737-754

Magill, J. (2009) *'It's hard to recognise the agile man I married'; Judith Magill's retirement dreams were dashed by her husband's Parkinson's disease Times Newspaper September 21.p.8*

McCall, B. (2006) *Living with Parkinson's Disease* Sheldon Press

MacLennan, W.J. (1998) Caring for Carers *Age and Aging* 1998; 27:651-652 [Online] Available from http://www.aging.oxfordjournals.org [Accessed 26 October 2010]

Macniven, J. (2009) *Psychological services for people with Parkinson's disease:* British Psychological Society

Martinez-Martin, P., Benito-Leon, J., Alonso, F., Catalan, J., Pondal, M., Zamarbide, I., Tobias, A. and de Pedro, J. (2005) quality of life of caregivers in Parkinson's disease *Qual life Res* (2005) 14: 463-472

Miller, E., Berrios, G. E. And Politynska, B. E. (1996) caring For Someone With Parkinson's Disease: Factors That Contribute to

Distress *International Journal of Geriatric Psychiatry.* Volume 11: 263-268 (1996)

Nettleton, S. (2006) *The Sociology of Health and Illness* 2nd Ed. Polity.

Ogden, J. (2007) *Health Psychology A Textbook* 4th ed. McGraw-Hill Open University Press.

O'Reilly, F., Finnan, F., Allwright, S., Smith, G.D. and Ben-Shlomo, Y. (1996) The effects of caring for a spouse with Parkinson's disease on social, psychological and physical well-being *British Journal of General Practice* 1996, 46, 507-512

Oxtoby, M., McCall, B. and Williams, A. (2004) *Parkinson's*: London; Class Publishing.

Parkinson's UK (2008) *Life with Parkinson's today – room for improvement: Results of the UK"s largest ever survey of people with Parkinson's and carers.* London: Parkinson's Disease Society.

Pentland, B. (1999) The nature and course of Parkinson's disease. In Percival, R. and Hobson, P. Eds. *Parkinson's Disease: Studies in Psychological and Social Care*: BPS Books. PP1-12

Reno, J. (2007) 'takes on Parkinson's disease with curiosity, not fear' *The Orange County Register*, April 24 [on-line] Available at:

http://articles.ocregister.com/2007-04-23/life/24678763_1_tremor-dyskinesia-parkinson-s-disease [Accessed 1st April 2010]

Schapira, T. (2006) *Understanding Parkinson's disease* : BMA Family doctor Books

Schrag, A., Ben-Shalono, Y. and Quinn, N. P. (2000) Cross-sectional prevalence study of idiopathic Parkinson's disease and Parkinsonism in London *British Medical Journal* 321, 21-22

Schrag, A., Hovris, A., Morley, D., Quinn, N. And Jahanshahi, M. (2006) Caregiver-burden in Parkinson's disease is closely associated with psychiatric symptoms, falls, and disability *Parkinsonism and related disorders* 12 (2006) 35-41 [on-line] Available from http://www.elsevier.com/locate/parkreldis [date accessed 26 0ctober 2010]

Secker, D. L. and Brown, R. G. (2005) Cognitive behavioural therapy (CBT) for carer's of patients with Parkinson's disease: a preliminary randomised controlled trial *J Neurol Neurosurg Psychiatry 2005;* 76: 491-497

Shroyer, J. and Dickinson, J. (1999) Ways to reduce the risk of falling in the home environment In Hutton, T. J. and Dippel, R. L. (1999) *Caring for the Parkinson's Patient*: Eds. Prometheus Books

Simon, C. ,Kumar, S. and Kendrick, T. (2002) Who cares for the carers? The district nurse perspective *Family Practice*: Volume 19 No1 Oxford University Press 2002 [on-line]

Spliethoff-Kamminga, N. G. A., Zwinderman, A.H., Springer, M.P. and Roos, R. A. (2003) A disease specific psychosocial questionnaire for Parkinson's disease caregivers *J Neurol* (2003) 250: 1162-1168

Stokes, A. (2010) *The caring reality of family carers*: [on-line] Available at: http://www.carealliance.ie/pdfs/FullReportFinal.pdf [Accessed] 15 January 2011

Vitaliano, P. P., Zhang, J. and Scanlan, J.M. (2003) Is care-giving hazardous to One's Health? *Psychological Bulletin* 2003, Vol. 129, No. 6, 946-972 [on-line] Available at:-

http://www.apa.org/pubs/journals/releases/bul-1296946.pdf Accessed 29 December 2010

Weiner, W. J., Shulman, L.M. and Lang, A. E. (2001) *Parkinson's disease A complete guide for Patients and families*: The John Hopkins University Press.

Williams, S. and Keady, J. (2008) A stony road...a 19 year journey: Bridging through late stage Parkinson's disease *Journal of*

Research in Nursing 2008 13: 373 [on-line] Available from
http://jm.sagepub.com/content/13/5/373 [Date accessed] 26
October 2010

World Health Organisation (1998) *Parkinson's disease: A unique
survey launched* Geneva: World Health Organisation

Worley, K. B. and Dippel, R.L. (1999) Parkinson's disease and the
family. In Hutton, T. J. and Dippel, R. L. (1999) *Caring for the
Parkinson's Patient*: Eds. Prometheus Books